PRA
THE INNOVA1

MW00414626

"This book had me hooked immediately. It covers all the bases and fills a void in the nursing leadership space. It is a must read for all nurses (and others) in a healthcare leadership role. I love the andragogical approach. Well done Dr. Clipper!"

–Michael Ackerman, PhD, RN, FCCM, FNAP, FAANP, FAAN
Clinical Professor
Director of Master of Healthcare Innovation Program
The Ohio State University College of Nursing

THE INNOVATION HANDBOOK

A NURSE LEADER'S GUIDE TO TRANSFORMING NURSING

BONNIE CLIPPER
DNP, MA, MBA, RN, CENP, FACHE, FAAN

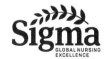

Sigma
GLOBAL NURSING
EXCELLENCE

Sigma Theta Tau International Honor Society of Nursing (Sigma) is a nonprofit organization whose mission is developing nurse leaders anywhere to improve healthcare everywhere. Founded in 1922, Sigma has more than 135,000 active members in over 100 countries and territories. Members include practicing nurses, instructors, researchers, policymakers, entrepreneurs, and others. Sigma's more than 540 chapters are located at more than 700 institutions of higher education throughout Armenia, Australia, Botswana, Brazil, Canada, Chile, Colombia, Croatia, England, Eswatini, Finland, Ghana, Hong Kong, Ireland, Israel, Italy, Jamaica, Japan, Jordan, Kenya, Lebanon, Malawi, Mexico, the Netherlands, Nigeria, Pakistan, Philippines, Portugal, Puerto Rico, Scotland, Singapore, South Africa, South Korea, Sweden, Taiwan, Tanzania, Thailand, the United States, and Wales. Learn more at www.sigmanursing.org.

Sigma Theta Tau International
550 West North Street
Indianapolis, IN, USA 46202

To request a review copy for course adoption, order additional books, buy in bulk, or purchase for corporate use, contact Sigma Marketplace at 888.654.4968 (US/Canada toll-free), +1.317.687.2256 (International), or solutions@sigmamarketplace.org.

To request author information, or for speaker or other media requests, contact Sigma Marketing at 888.634.7575 (US/Canada toll-free) or +1.317.634.8171 (International).

ISBN: 9781646480784
EPUB ISBN: 9781646480791
PDF ISBN: 9781646480814
MOBI ISBN: 9781646481187

LCCN: 2023009111

First Printing, 2023

Publisher: Dustin Sullivan   **Managing Editor:** Carla Hall
Acquisitions Editor: Emily Hatch   **Publications Specialist:** Todd Lothery
Development Editor: Kate Shoup   **Proofreader:** Jane Palmer
Cover Designer: Rebecca Batchelor **Interior Design/Layout:** Rebecca Batchelor
Indexer: Larry Sweazy

DEDICATION

This book is dedicated to my two kids, Sean and Ella. I find joy and purpose in making the world a better place for their future, and health and healthcare are part of that. I believe that one can do good and do well, and my goal is to create an impactful life—for me, for them, for all of us.

ACKNOWLEDGMENTS

Thank you to my friends and nurse colleagues who graciously shared their wisdom and insights, which are peppered throughout the book. I am forever grateful to all nurses who do the difficult work of providing patient care. The world owes you a big debt of gratitude, and nurse leaders owe you a safer and easier way to do what you love. Nurses and nurse leaders are the inspiration for my work to transform nursing and to motivate positive deviants everywhere!

ABOUT THE AUTHOR

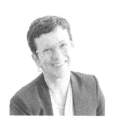

Bonnie Clipper, DNP, MA, MBA, RN, CENP, FACHE, FAAN, is a former healthcare executive. After more than 20 years as a chief nurse executive, Clipper founded Innovation Advantage. She was also the first Vice President of Innovation at the American Nurses Association, where she created an innovation strategy to draw more than 4 million nurses into the innovation space.

An internationally recognized nurse futurist, Clipper was a coauthor of the seminal work *The Innovation Roadmap: A Guide for Nurse Leaders*. She was also the lead author of the international best-selling book *The Nurse's Guide to Innovation*. Clipper regularly publishes and blogs on technologies affecting nursing. She is the sole nurse member of the HIMSS Innovation Board of Advisors and is a startup coach for MATTER, a global health tech accelerator.

Clipper earned her bachelor of science degree in nursing from Winona State University, her master of arts (leadership) degree from St. Mary's University, her master of business administration degree from Lewis University, and her doctorate in nursing leadership from Texas Tech University Health Sciences Center. Clipper is an RWJF Executive Nurse Fellow alumna, an ASU/AONL Executive Fellow in Innovative Health Leadership alumna, and a fellow in the American Academy of Nursing. She enjoys 21st-century problem-solving and is a top healthcare influencer, nurse futurist, podcast host, and global speaker.

ADDITIONAL BOOK RESOURCES

For a sample chapter and other book-related resources, follow the link or QR code below.

https://sigma.nursingrepository.org/handle/10755/23090

TABLE OF CONTENTS

FOREWORD

How many of you have been in this scenario? After months of planning, you are finally at your organization's innovation event. Dozens, maybe hundreds, of you have assembled, fully caffeinated and crumbling pastry in hand. Today is the day you solve the biggest problems in healthcare.

The morning starts off with a powerful keynote from the leadership team framing the opportunities and encouraging you to be bold, challenge the status quo, and think outside the box. You are revved up, split into teams, and asked to fill out colorful Post-It notes with ideas. Ideas flow from your pen as your excitement builds to share them with your table. The rest of the room is in a flurry of conversation, coffee refills, and "innovation."

A short time later, you begin to place your Post-It ideas on the wall, and inevitably, the lumpers and splitters emerge from the crowd. Clumping ideas together, splitting out subgroups, turning 3×3-inch square papers into a work of art in front of your very eyes. Next, the facilitator comes along and hands out colored, sticky dots so you can "vote" on the ideas. After a tense five minutes, the dot votes are in: Idea #1 got 26 votes, and idea #2 got 14 votes. You have a clear winner! Afterward, while the room enjoys a well-deserved pizza lunch, the facilitator walks around the room, taking pictures of all the Post-Its, ideas, and people for the website.

This is not innovation.

What you just experienced is a Post-It note pizza party. You came to the room unprepared, gave out lots of opinions based on your current knowledge base, arbitrarily voted on these ideas, and selected a "winner." That is not how innovation works—yet organization after organization does this every year.

Innovation is a rigorous process backed by data, science, and method that is intended to solve challenging problems with unknown solutions. Innovation requires processes, time, resources, evidence, and leadership as well as brainstorming and energy. The problem is that very few people in healthcare have taken the time to learn the science of change and innovation. The result is that Post-It noting and dot voting become the manifestations of innovation. It's a box to check rather than a culture that is cultivated. While there is value in prioritizing new ideas, the process of innovation takes more preparation.

For nursing and healthcare to evolve through its current paradigm-shifting moment, we need more nurses and clinicians, more leaders, and more organizations to understand and utilize the science and tactics of true innovation. This is why I am excited to see *The Innovation Handbook: A Nurse Leader's Guide to Transforming Nursing*, by Bonnie Clipper. This leader's guide to innovation will be a key resource to help our teams innovate and ultimately transform the way we do things. There is value in using a rigorous process of innovation combined with powerful tools. Together these can elicit new thinking to transform nursing and healthcare and start solving real problems. Most importantly, do something!

–Dan Weberg, PhD, MHI, RN, FAAN

INTRODUCTION

---- **"** ----

"Change is the law of life. And those who look only to the past or present are certain to miss the future."

–John F. Kennedy

---- **,,** ----

Welcome to *The Innovation Handbook: A Nurse Leader's Guide to Transforming Nursing.* I am thrilled you are reading this book. I realize there are many books in this space, and I am grateful that you chose this one.

The healthcare ecosystem is in a state of chaos. We have never seen the level of disruption and turnover that we are seeing now. It is in desperate need of true transformation. The same is true for the nursing profession.

As nurses, we must be the ones to drive new models of care delivery, create novel roles, and integrate technologies to provide the care and outcomes our patients and communities need. Engaging in thoughtful and respectful conversations about scheduling, staffing, value-based care, nursing reimbursement, outcome tracking, and more is something that every nurse must do, however difficult that might be. Watching from the sidelines and making negative comments about our profession, colleagues, and patients as an anonymous social media user is not only *not* OK—it diminishes the credibility and importance of our profession.

It is time to lean in to create a better future for nursing and for healthcare overall. Imagine the power of leaders and direct-care nurses working to transform their own practice or organization!

We would be unstoppable—leading the way to solve some of the most vexing challenges of our time. Let's use our status as the most trusted profession to accomplish great things.

This book is not intended to be a theory-heavy textbook. There are already a few of those on the market (and they are all fantastic). Rather, it's meant to be a "how to" manual or toolkit. It's intended to be a practical guide and toolkit to enlighten nurse leaders and inform their transformation as we work to solve this crisis. It takes a scrappy, pragmatic approach to provide you with a foundation of knowledge, to give you ideas, and to challenge you as a leader to apply the concepts and think differently. I want you to take notes in it, highlight passages, dog-ear pages, and carry it around in your bag of choice.

There are data in this book that may at times feel unfavorable and even contrary. I've included these data to provoke you, to push you, and to generate a call to action. Transforming nursing and healthcare will require all of us working to create change—and quickly. This book is meant to convey this sense of urgency. Having said that, there are times when going fast in the long-term means moving slowly and methodically in the short term, and this book reflects that too.

The ideal readers for this book are nurse leaders at all levels—including charge nurses, managers, directors, and nurse executives—who are hoping to find inspiration, nuggets of insight, or new ways of thinking about old problems. It doesn't matter if you have years of experience or are new to your role. Learning why we need to change, thinking about ways to change, and becoming a champion of change are all important, for all of us. Leading successful change is a numbers game. We need more trained leaders and direct care nurses with an innovative skill set to accomplish our goals. We are all students of change!

For nurse leaders, these are chaotic times. It can be difficult to remain optimistic. But we don't have to accept the current state of affairs. With the right skills, we can create a future that works for us. Now more than ever, we need to align and collaborate. We must help each other innovate to improve care delivery. We must transform nursing into a more forward-thinking profession, and we must do it together.

In this book, I have identified concepts that I believe will help you become a more innovative leader. I approached writing this book by reflecting on what would have helped me as a nurse leader looking for ways to think differently and to experiment with novel approaches, with the goal of enticing you to join the effort to transform our profession. No book is perfect, this one included, but I believe it will help you start on your personal innovation journey. I hope everyone who reads this book will learn something new and will apply it to make their practice ecosystem better than it was before.

This book flows in a way that is intended to help you connect the dots and generate your own innovative ideas along the way. Each chapter kicks off with a brief preview of what you can expect to take away from that chapter. It also lists objectives. These are clues to target your learning and provide specific ways to put new concepts into action while building your innovation competencies. Various sections in each chapter cover concepts, definitions, ideas, tools, and frameworks to provide a foundation for your innovation practice and build your innovation skill set. You'll see call-out boxes from nurse experts throughout the book that provide insights and different points of view. You'll also find notes and tips sprinkled throughout the book to accelerate your pace of learning and your innovation journey. The overall goal of the book is to inform you, engage you, and challenge you to solve real, deep-rooted problems in your organization, community, or region, or even at a national level.

I want *all* of us to work together to transform systems and modernize nursing practice. Achieving this enormous goal, however, will start with small steps. The first of these is to build competency as a change agent. From there, we can develop broad innovation practices and hopefully attain transformation. Transformation is the pinnacle of change. It's difficult to achieve and even harder to sustain. Don't just dabble in transformation. Running a hackathon or other innovation event every so often won't do. For transformation, you must go all in. I am counting on you to transform nursing!

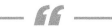

"If you want to go fast go alone, if you want to go far, go together."

–African Proverb

With gratitude,
Bonnie Clipper, DNP, MA, MBA, RN, CENP, FACHE, FAAN

P.S. If you develop your own innovative practices and ideas, don't hesitate to share them with me! You can find me on LinkedIn at https://www.linkedin.com/in/bonnieclipper/.

"I am of certain convinced that the greatest heroes are those who do their duty in the daily grind of domestic affairs whilst the world whirls as a maddening dreidel."

—Florence Nightingale

CHAPTER 1

The Current State of Nursing and the Need to Transform

KEYWORDS

Nursing economics, nursing shortage, nursing workforce data, workforce challenge

This chapter serves to "level set" by highlighting facts about the current, unsustainable state of nursing. It discusses the need for transformation, the importance of developing new and innovative competencies, and how these can be leveraged to transform nursing at a time that requires urgency and a drastically different approach.

OBJECTIVES

- Describe the nursing supply and demand-based production model and ways to increase the supply of nurses in the future.

- Identify novel ideas to improve the long-term retention of new graduate nurses.

Nursing as a profession has existed since 1854, when Florence Nightingale "formalized" the work of caregiving in her occupation as a caretaker of soldiers during the Crimean War. While Nightingale wasn't necessarily the first nurse, she is one of the most influential. A prolific writer, she kept meticulous notes and journals and created processes and systems for how care should be delivered (Riegel et al., 2021). Her foresight provided a sound foundation for our profession to develop and evolve upon.

Now, however, we are far beyond what even Nightingale envisioned. The healthcare world in which we practice today is much more complex and dynamic than she could have ever dreamed of. It is important for us, as leaders, to understand our history and traditions and to use these as a springboard to advance our work of incorporating evidence, innovation, and even entrepreneurship into our transformation. Otherwise, we run the risk of being stuck in the age of Nightingale and becoming irrelevant.

> Transformation is essential for our profession to survive and thrive in the future. This will be driven by our ability to dream big and innovate.

Much like the rest of the healthcare ecosystem, the practice of nursing continues to rapidly evolve. At times, it feels as though it is spinning out of control. Over the years, nurses have become much more specialized, which is to be expected given the complexity of patient care and practices that we employ to improve patient outcomes. Today, there are 183 specialty certifications in nursing (Nurse.org, 2021) accompanied by more than 100 national and international high-level professional organizations (not including the state-level and regional-level chapters of many of these organizations; Nurse.org, n.d.). Often, there is little (if any) alignment in what many of these organizations espouse or support, nor is there consistent alignment across the nursing industry as a whole. Thus, our profession suffers from confusion and the lack of a consistent message to address the complexity, causes, and solutions of the current workforce situation.

The stress and difficulties of the current nursing environment cannot be overstated. The impact of retirements, burnout, the COVID-19 pandemic, violence in the workplace, career opportunities for nurses in other industries, and other problems on what is already a chaotic, life-or-death industry cannot be overstated. This has created a nearly untenable practice environment for the nation's 4.3 million nurses (American Nurses Association, n.d.). This must change—and nurses are the ones who must change it.

"Technology innovation combined with the changing healthcare landscape will expand nursing practice to include diverse settings and venues. These settings include retail pharmacies, community services, genomics, home care standards, digital technology roles, and payers. The roles are now hybrid, where nurses will use skill sets from different domains: informatics, technology tools, research, and value-based purchasing. Advances in technology are radically changing the employment landscape. The nursing workforce will become more complex and faster-moving than ever. We need to change how we educate future nurses and, as a byproduct of care delivery, measure our impact on outcomes showing value to the bottom line."

–Rosemary Kennedy, PhD, MBA, RN, FAAN

HIGH-LEVEL WORKFORCE CHALLENGES

Challenges facing the nursing profession are internal as well as external, and financial as well as regulatory in nature. And of course, many of them have been decades in the making. To identify solutions to the problems facing nurses today, we need to start by honestly talking about the challenges we face. These challenges help explain the high turnover rates among nurses, which contributes to and compounds the nursing shortage. They include the following:

- Inadequate staffing

- Unsafe work environments from a practice perspective

- Concerns about compensation

- Lack of a value-based reimbursement model for nursing services

> Just to be clear, the COVID-19 pandemic did *not* cause the turnover trajectory in nursing. It simply accelerated and exacerbated what was already in progress.

- Scheduling and work-life balance

- Incivility and bullying from colleagues in the workplace

- Violence in the workplace from patients, families, and even colleagues

- Workload and lack of support resources

- Difficulty in building a workforce pipeline

- Lack of capacity and faculty shortages in nursing schools

- Employment opportunities for nurses (internal and external to healthcare)

A variety of surveys over the past few years identified many of these same challenges. Table 1.1 shows the top challenges cited by nurses in two different surveys, administered by two different groups over one year apart, despite notable differences among these data sets (including differences related to the COVID-19 pandemic).

Table 1.1   *Issues Affecting Nurses: A Comparison*

Advisory Board (2021)	American Nurses Foundation (2022a)
Insufficient staffing levels	Insufficient staffing
Intensity of workload	N/A
Emotional toll of the job	Work negatively affecting health/ wellbeing
Not feeling supported	Lack of support from their employer during the pandemic
The physical toll of the job	Distrust of my employer
Seeking higher-paid positions	Need for higher income
Insufficient personal protective equipment (due to COVID-19 pandemic)	Poor organizational response to COVID-19 pandemic

As a profession, our current path is unsustainable. There simply are not enough people who are either already practicing nurses or in the process of becoming nurses to meet the projected demand (which is based on how we currently use nurses). There will always be patients, but if there are not enough nurses, who will care for them? Rest assured, someone will—but that someone might be a new type of provider practicing a new discipline, or perhaps part of a new cadre of unlicensed personnel. One potential solution

Although none of these lists are comprehensive, it is easy to see some consistent themes and recurring trends.

now being tossed about is "lowering the bar" in terms of who is qualified to become a nurse. This seems rather unwise, however, as we may rapidly find ourselves dealing with a slew of entirely new challenges associated with poor outcomes due to lack of competence.

This is why it is so important for nurses to be involved in addressing their issues and driving these conversations. We as nurses must confront our many challenges and work to improve and save our profession. We must lead the discussion on transforming care-delivery models, leveraging technology in nursing practice, developing nursing reimbursement models, reimagining the nursing education pipeline, and so on. Nurses cannot do this alone, however. CEOs, CFOs, other executives, physicians, hospital boards, deans, unions, and anyone even peripherally related to the nursing profession must commit to addressing these challenges. This is often a problem, however, due to politics, competition, or unaligned interests. Simply throwing money at these problems won't work—not now and not in the long term. Too many processes and systems are simply broken or outdated.

As a first step, it's important to review data so we understand why it is so urgent for us as nurses to transform our own profession and practice. This means becoming aware of trends associated with topics such as turnover rates, salaries, demographics, supply and demand by region, leader trends, education data, and so on. Fortunately, accurate data and reliable reports are readily available that provide some insight into the current state of nursing. For example:

- **The Bureau of Labor Statistics Occupational Outlook Handbook for Registered Nurses:** https://www.bls.gov/ooh/healthcare/registered-nurses.htm

- **NSI National Health Care & RN Retention Survey:** https://www.nsinursingsolutions.com/Documents/Library/NSI_National_Health_Care_Retention_Report.pdf

- **McKinsey Insights on Healthcare Systems & Services:** https://www.mckinsey.com/industries/healthcare-systems-and-services/our-insights

- **American Nurses Foundation and American Nurses Association COVID-19 Survey Series Results:** https://www.nursingworld.org/practice-policy/work-environment/health-safety/disaster-preparedness/coronavirus/what-you-need-to-know/survey-series-results/

- **American Association of Colleges of Nursing Snapshot of Today's Nursing Workforce:** https://www.aacnnursing.org/News-Information/Nursing-Shortage-Resources/Workforce

> Data don't lie, although there may be more than one way of interpreting them.

NURSING SUPPLY

Data on turnover and vacancy rates in nursing represent a five-alarm fire. There is no doubt that the nursing landscape is changing rapidly. When you envision the nursing workforce pipeline as a supply and demand-based production model, think of it as a scale or child's teeter-totter. There are supply *inputs* (nurses entering the profession) and impacts on the supply or demand, simplified as *outputs* (nurses leaving the profession). (See Figure 1.1.) In an overly simplified way, there should be some homeostasis, equity, or parity in the movement on both ends of the scale to attain an adequate supply of nurses in the workforce.

INPUTS = OUTPUTS
(nurses entering the profession)   (nurses leaving the profession)

FIGURE 1.1   A simplified view of the nursing workforce pipeline.

To provide some context, based on data from the last 10 years, we knew we would experience a nursing shortage in the future. What has changed in the last three years is that the shortage that has already begun is projected to worsen. By 2025 we are expected to have a deficit of between 200,000 and 450,000 direct care nurses—a shortfall of 10 to 20% (Berlin et al., 2022).

Nurses Are Not a Commodity

Some people suggest we are *not* in a nursing shortage, but rather are experiencing a redistribution problem. While we might talk about producing nurses or supply-and-demand challenges, nurses are not commodities that can easily be moved from one region to another. Nurses are people with families. They have partners with jobs, children in school, and community connections. Thinking of nursing as a commodity is one of the largest threats to nursing as a profession today.

To understand the data behind our staffing concerns, let's begin with turnover data. According to a 2022 survey conducted on 272 hospitals, with more than 166,000 registered nurses responding, national direct-care nurse turnover is reported to be 27.1% (NSI Nursing Solutions, 2022, p. 4). Moreover, the trends are not favorable, demonstrating a year-over-year increase when compared to another survey that indicates that average RN turnover rate in 2020 was 18.6% and 16.9% in 2019 (Advisory Board, 2021).

As for vacancy rates, in 2021, the Advisory Board stated that 35.8% of hospitals reported a vacancy rate of 10% or greater, compared to 23.9% of hospitals in 2019 (Advisory Board, 2021). Another survey found the national average RN vacancy rate was 17.0%—7.1 points higher than 2021 (NSI Nursing Solutions, 2022, p. 1).

New Graduate Nurse Turnover

Data concerning turnover, or *churn*, among new graduate nurses are especially troubling. In 2019, the turnover rate of nurses with less than one year of experience was 24%, and in 2020, this increased slightly to 24.6% (Advisory Board, 2021). It wasn't until 2021 that the impact of an increasingly chaotic practice environment and the COVID-19 pandemic demonstrated their influence on new nurses, however. A 2021 survey found that new graduate nurses had a turnover rate of approximately 18 to 30% within their first 12 months employed as a nurse, and 34 to 57% within their first 24 months (Advisory Board, 2021). Meanwhile, a 2022 survey found that 31% of all newly hired RNs left within their first year, with first-year turnover accounting for more than a quarter (27.7%) of all RN turnover (NSI Nursing Solutions, 2022, p. 10). In this survey, it is not clear that "newly hired RNs" refers to new graduate nurses. Still, at this rate, within three years, the average organization could turn over all of their newly hired graduate nurses.

A 2021 survey revealed that two years is now the average amount of time a newly graduated nurse spends at the bedside before leaving their role, although it is uncertain as to whether these nurses are leaving nursing entirely or just leaving their current organization (Advisory Board, 2021). An analysis of nurses who work at EPIC (electronic health record) facilities reveals another perspective: Across the country, nurse tenure decreased from 3.6 years to 2.78 years for nurses working 12-hour shifts between March 2021 and March 2022. These data also show that median tenure dropped in the West by 32.2%, compared to 11.3% in the South, 16.4% in the Midwest, and 17.7% in the Northeast (Thayer et al., 2022).

To compound these concerns, a June 2022 analysis of 400,000 nurses accompanied by a survey of new graduate nurses identified that 55% of new graduate nurses plan to leave the nursing profession "prior to retirement." In other words, they do not plan to remain nurses for as long as previous generations of nurses did. According to the new graduate nurses, there are two main reasons for this: staffing shortages/high workload and ineffective onboarding/training leading to them feeling unsafe in their practice (Abuzeid, 2022). All this highlights the fact that there is a high level of churn on the front end of the career spectrum, and fewer nurses will make it to the middle or late stage of their nursing careers.

The Need to Change the Tide

A 2022 survey of nearly 13,000 nurses conducted by the American Nurses Foundation revealed that 52% of nurses are considering or may consider leaving their current position (American Nurses Foundation, 2022b, p. 4). This compares to the previous year (2021) survey of nearly 23,000 nurses, in which 39% of nurses indicated they intended to leave or were considering leaving their current position (American Nurses Foundation, 2022a, p. 4).

The issue of turnover is more concerning when the data are segmented by age cohort. For example, 63% of nurses under the age of 35 indicated their intent/consideration of leaving. In comparison, of nurses in the 55 or older cohort, who are potentially nearing retirement, 43% intend to leave or are considering leaving their position (American Nurses Foundation, 2022b, p. 4). These data are supported by a 2021 survey in which 22% of direct care nurses indicated they may leave their current position within the next 12 months (Advisory Board, 2021). It is easy to see why these data and trends are concerning; they're simply unsustainable.

Don't despair. Not all of the news is bad. There are glimmers of hope and reasons to be optimistic. One major positive development is the exponential growth in the number of nurse practitioners. In fact, by 2030, experts project there will be 396,546 practicing nurse practitioners (Advisory Board, 2021), many of them members of Gen Z. This is incredibly encouraging! Let's learn from this and find ways to apply these lessons to address other workforce pipeline challenges.

Demand Projections

To better understand the need to urgently transform nursing, let's switch to a conversation about nursing demand projections. Think about what was discussed earlier regarding the inputs and the outputs, which focused on the supply side of this equation. Now think about the demand side of this model and the fact that registered nurse employment is projected to grow 9% from 2020 to 2030 (US Bureau of Labor Statistics, 2022); this indicates increased demand. To further expand on the demand side of the equation, the Bureau of Labor Statistics projects approximately 194,500 openings for registered nurses per year for the next 10 years, with the majority of these openings due to turnover and retirement. A survey in 2021 found that healthcare vacancies will continue to increase in 2022, with 62% of hospitals planning to grow their labor force and 64% of hospitals indicating that they are planning to expand their RN employee base (NSI Nursing Solutions, 2022, p. 12). With demand for nurses increasing and supply of nurses decreasing, think about how we can resolve the mismatch.

Meanwhile, while nursing school applications have increased slightly, the American Association of Colleges of Nursing highlights our struggle to keep up with demand in the report 2021–2022 *Enrollment and Graduations in Baccalaureate and Graduate Programs in Nursing*, where the data indicate that in 2021, US nursing schools declined entry to 91,938 qualified applications from baccalaureate and graduate nursing programs due to the "insufficient number of faculty, clinical sites, classroom space, and clinical preceptors, as well as budget constraints" (American Association of Colleges of Nursing, 2022, p. 2). This is an obvious part of the supply side of the workforce pipeline that needs to be immediately addressed through a plethora of creative solutions.

NURSING OUTCOMES

The impact of churn on direct care nurses (as well as their leaders) cannot be overstated. It is constantly discussed on social media, in news articles—even between friends and family. It seems as though everyone has (or knows someone who has) a story of how they were affected by significant staffing shortages.

One of the most profound and upsetting impacts of this is its impact on the wellbeing of individual nurses and their subsequent burnout. During the COVID-19 pandemic, nurses were originally lauded as heroes, but things took a turn about midway through. Now, more than two years after the onset of COVID-19, nurses rate their mental health at an average score of 5.8, compared to a pre-pandemic score of 7.8—a 26% decline. Meanwhile, 75% of those surveyed report feeling burned out (TrustedHealth, 2022, pp. 4–5). The workplace has also changed dramatically. A January 2022 survey by the American Nurses Foundation of 11,964 nurses showed that 60% reported experiences of bullying/incivility at work, with the majority of these coming from patients and their families (American Nurses Foundation, 2022b).

Impact on Patient Care

Every week, we see headlines about the effect of the nursing shortage on nurses' mental wellbeing and its direct impact on patient care. One interesting outcome of high nurse turnover highlighted a growing new concern: the experience-complexity gap. This illustrates the widening gap between the experience level of nurses at the bedside and the complexity of patient care acuity (Virkstis et al., 2019).

As nurses of the baby boomer generation continue to retire and we lose their many years of experience and organizational knowledge, we are faced with a growing lack of skills and knowledge. Increasing patient acuity, more complicated care, and more complex care delivery have resulted in a gap between nurses' skills and patients' care needs. This gap between nurses' skills and level of experience and the complexity of patients will have a direct impact on patient care, safety, and outcomes.

Economic Impact

On the financial side, we are seeing a dramatic increase in the cost of labor, mostly due to the need for contract labor or agency nursing staff to fill vacancies or to supplement existing staff.

In 2022, the average cost of turnover for a direct care RN was $46,100 (NSI Nursing Solutions, 2022). To take that one step further, a "one percent change in RN turnover will cost/save an average hospital an additional $262,300 per year" (NSI Nursing Solutions, 2022, p. 4).

To further expand on the economic impact, in 2021, it was projected that the inpatient revenue lost for a 300- to 500-bed hospital is approximately $90,000 per day when that hospital is understaffed (Advisory Board, 2021). However, we also know that to replace the actual work the nurse does through the use of internal premium or external contract labor is multiples higher. For example, travel nurse rates recently spiked over 200%, with contract labor averaging $154 per hour; moreover, for a short time, the top end of the hourly rate range was $225 per hour (NSI Nursing Solutions, 2022, p. 12). This does not include bonuses or free housing. Numbers like this grab the attention of financial executives every time.

"Train people well enough so they can leave, treat them well enough so they won't want to."

−Sir Richard Branson

CONCLUSION

The impact of industry-wide staffing shortages on nurses' mental health and overall wellbeing, not to mention patient care and the cost of labor, is enormous. As was highlighted in this chapter, for a variety of reasons, there are not enough people to meet today's needs for patient care, nor will there be enough nurses in the future. The math is not in our favor. This is why we are at the critical juncture of disruption and must take up the call to be innovative and to transform nursing. It is time to get out of our own heads, get out of our own way, and get to work. There are not 2, 10, 20, or even 100 solutions to the problems that now plague the nursing profession. Rather, transforming the nursing workforce and the delivery of care will require a multitude of incremental and disruptive innovations.

REFERENCES

Abuzeid, I. (2022, June 15). *New nurses are already planning to quit.* https://www.incrediblehealth.com/blog/new-nurse-study/

Advisory Board. (2021). *Hard truths for CNOs: The current and future state of the nursing workforce.* [PowerPoint Slides]. Advisory Board Nursing Executive Center National Meeting.

American Association of Colleges of Nursing. (2022, October). *Fact sheet: Nursing shortage.* https://www.aacnnursing.org/Portals/42/News/Factsheets/Nursing-Shortage-Factsheet.pdf

American Nurses Association. (n.d.). *Nurses in the workforce.* https://www.nursingworld.org/practice-policy/workforce/

American Nurses Foundation. (2022a, March 1). *Pulse on the nation's nurses survey series: COVID-19 two-year impact assessment survey.* https://www.nursingworld.org/~492857/contentassets/872ebb13c63f44f6b11a1bd0c74907c9/covid-19-two-year-impact-assessment-written-report-final.pdf

American Nurses Foundation. (2022b, January). COVID-19 impact assessment survey – the second year. https://www.nursingworld.org/practice-policy/work-environment/health-safety/disaster-preparedness/coronavirus/what-you-need-to-know/covid-19-impact-assessment-survey---the-second-year/

Berlin, G., Lapointe, M., Murphy, M., & Wexler, J. (2022, May 11). *Assessing the lingering impact of COVID-19 on the nursing workforce.* McKinsey & Company. https://www.mckinsey.com/industries/healthcare/our-insights/assessing-the-lingering-impact-of-covid-19-on-the-nursing-workforce

NSI Nursing Solutions. (2022). *2022 NSI national health care retention & RN staffing report.* https://www.nsinursingsolutions.com/Documents/Library/NSI_National_Health_Care_Retention_Report.pdf

Nurse.org. (n.d.). *List of nursing organizations.* https://nurse.org/orgs.shtml

Nurse.org. (2021, December 1). *Complete list of common nursing certifications.* https://nurse.org/articles/nursing-certifications-credentials-list/

Riegel, F., Crossetti, M. G. O., Martini, J. G., & Nes, A. A, G. (2021). Florence Nightingale's theory and her contributions to holistic critical thinking in nursing. *Revista Brasileira de Enfermagem,* 74(2), 1–5. https://www.scielo.br/j/reben/a/hLkJwbxtP5hGFPJSpzP9RMd/?format=pdf&lang=en

Thayer, J., Zillmer, J., Sandberg, N., Miller, A., Nagel, P., & MacGibbon, A. (2022, June 2). *'The new nurse' is the new normal.* Epic Research. https://epicresearch.org/articles/the-new-nurse-is-the-new-normal

Trusted Health. (2022). 2022 frontline nurse mental health & wellbeing survey. https://assets-global.website-files.com/62991a992ad4fe937e88efec/62d1ba32d9f1be54b8361503_Trusted%20Health%202022%20Mental%20Health%20Survey.pdf

US Bureau of Labor Statistics. (2022, September 8). *Registered nurses. Job outlook.* https://www.bls.gov/ooh/healthcare/registered-nurses.htm#tab-6

Virkstis, K., Herleth, A., & Rewers, L. (2019). Closing nursing's experience-complexity gap. *Journal of Nursing Administration,* 49(12), 580–582.

CHAPTER 2

Speaking the Same Language

KEYWORDS

Complex adaptive systems, complexity leadership, frameworks, innovation, positive deviance, transformation

This chapter provides definitions, concepts, and frameworks to ensure that leaders have a common language to inform their innovation- and transformation-related work. The definitions of innovation, improvement, and transformation, as well as knowns and unknowns, VUCA, complex adaptive systems, and complexity leadership, offer contextual platforms for the rapidly evolving healthcare ecosystem and help to level-set the work of transforming nursing and innovating to improve the healthcare paradigm.

OBJECTIVES

- Demonstrate appropriate use of terms necessary to innovate our way through the nursing crisis.

- Create a plan to educate colleagues and teams on the concepts shared in this chapter to increase the use of a common language for transformation.

When thinking about how to transform the current healthcare system and, more directly, the nursing profession, it is important that all involved speak the same language. To that end, this chapter covers standard concepts and definitions. A common nomenclature is essential to ensure alignment, promote a collective understanding, provide context for our transformation work, and allow greater influence in discussions pertaining to innovation. This is true among peers and colleagues as well as across hierarchical relationships and boundary-spanning roles.

HEALTHCARE SYSTEMS

Let's start by talking about *healthcare systems*. These systems have historically been viewed as large machines with clearly delineated boundaries, generally predictable outputs, and lateral or linear functions. However, due to the complexity of modern-day organizations, reimbursement, and delivery, healthcare systems have become much more complicated. This is also true of the healthcare ecosystem as a whole, which is now characterized by loose boundaries, a blurry or non-identifiable single locus of control, much less predictable outcomes, multiple relationships, complex dependencies, and matrixed or nonlinear functions (Petrie & Swanson, 2018). Leading transformative, large-scale, and sweeping change in this increasingly complex healthcare environment requires significant interpersonal and cognitive skill building (Petrie & Swanson, 2018).

IMPROVEMENT

Improvement generally involves an incremental and often iterative model, with different cycles compounding and building upon each other to optimize and reduce the number of defects within the existing system (Mate, 2017). Opportunities for improvement often lend themselves to questioning whether the problem is ripe for innovation instead. Improvement is often safer and easier than innovation, because we can already see what an improved version would look like, whereas innovation is likely unknown and untested. The result of an innovation is harder to imagine than how an improvement would pan out.

While improvement is generally iterative, innovation can be either incremental or truly transformative. When pondering whether to improve or innovate, consider whether the system in question can support small tweaks only or large transformational changes. The nursing profession would benefit from many incremental changes, but it is *really* ripe for broad, sweeping transformation.

Evaluating an Improvement or Innovation

Questions may arise when evaluating a possible improvement or innovation, such as:

- Where are the opportunities?
- Is it reducing variation?
- Is it eliminating waste?
- Is it reducing inefficiencies? (Weberg & Davidson, 2021)

INNOVATION

It seems like defining innovation should be pretty cut and dry. However, it's actually somewhat complex, because there are multiple definitions. In an interview with Johnson & Johnson (2018), nurse entrepreneur Wayne Nix said, "One of the biggest challenges of innovation is defining what it is." One well-known definition suggests that innovation in healthcare is "those changes that help healthcare practitioners focus on the patient by helping healthcare professionals work smarter, faster, better, and more cost-effectively" (Thaker et al., 2012, p. 364). Another definition—one of my favorites—is applying new ideas into practice or using existing ideas in new ways (Melynk & Davidson, 2009).

Building a culture of innovation starts with an organization's top leader. The highest-level executive in an organization must commit to any transformation effort for it to be successful, to be sustainable, and to provide the best outcomes. From there, innovative behaviors must trickle down to every single level in the organization's hierarchy and touch every person within the organization's ecosystem to encourage the necessary shift in mindset for both employees and leaders to truly become empowered innovators. This shift is incredibly powerful and can energize individuals even through simple acts, such as leaders asking team members about innovative work that is being done on the unit/department level and posing probing questions about goals and results when rounding.

> Leadership rounding without purpose or intent is basically just a walk through the facility.

All organizations like to believe that they are innovative. However, this is quite often not the case. While it is true that many—perhaps most—organizations have a spirit of innovation and a desire to innovate, few provide evidence of a culture of innovation. The bottom line is, an organization's culture must support a change in behavior that lends itself to innovation. The organization must create a culture in which innovation and transformation are not only encouraged but *expected*. In addition, support and resources must be in place for

> Many organizations that believe they *are* innovative really aren't.

individuals and teams to successfully align their journey with this *expectation*. Otherwise, innovation within the organization cannot occur (Weberg & Davidson, 2021).

Crucially, innovation within an organization isn't happenstance or serendipitous. Rather, it is intentional, focused, and sustained. One hackathon or other innovation-oriented event per year isn't enough. While these may be catalysts and often energize the organization, *true* innovation requires far more rigor and ongoing and intentional effort.

Seeking Inspiration for Innovation Outside the Healthcare Arena

Many healthcare providers believe that there are too many risks and too many unknowns to allow for innovation. We also believe that unless you're in healthcare, you don't understand how things work, so there's no way you can help us fix things. This is particularly true among nurses. We are not very receptive to outside voices. Unfortunately, this has kept us in a closed system of thought and ignorant of the possibilities, and it has become an impediment for us to move our profession forward.

It is time to look outside healthcare for answers. Whether it's the aviation industry, the supply chain industry, the tech industry, or something else entirely, we must learn how other industries have successfully innovated to improve their workflows, accomplish their goals, and transform their professions.

Technology companies often have great frameworks for innovating, typically involving *design thinking* (discussed later in this book). Technology companies also tend to have a flatter organizational structure to allow ideas to bubble up from employees to top executives. Google famously instituted what it called the "20% time rule," which encouraged employees, "in addition to their regular projects, to spend 20% of their time working on what they think will most benefit Google" (Murphy, 2020, p. 1) The healthcare industry could learn from these practices!

On a related note, a 2022 study revealed that 25% of the total cost of healthcare—equal to $265 billion—will shift fee-for-service Medicare and Medicare Advantage beneficiaries from inpatient to home-based care (Bestsennyy et al., 2022, para. 2). Meanwhile, more and more nurse practitioners are being employed by telehealth companies, retail chains such as CVS and Walmart, and online outlets like Amazon. Both of these shifts suggest that although the majority of nurses now work in inpatient acute-care hospitals, that won't be the case for long. And many companies entering the healthcare market are billion-dollar corporations that value innovation—meaning there will soon be an even higher demand for innovative approaches to care. This provides an excellent opportunity for the nursing profession to transform how we train, use, and deploy nurses using ideas from outside the healthcare arena.

POSITIVE DEVIANCE

Positive deviance describes the "intentional act of breaking the rules in order to serve the greater good" (Gary, 2013, p. 26). Moreover, positive deviance is "often viewed as a process or approach to organizational change, or as a framework for understanding organizational behaviors; as an alternative method of identifying best practices; as a valuable tool for identifying innovative healthcare practices; and as a problem-solving technique" (Gary, 2013, p. 28). While there is an element of risk to the person who is doing the deviating, positive deviance it is generally "well-intentioned and can revolve around adapting, creating or innovation to meet the needs of the situation" (Gary, 2013, p. 26).

Positive deviance occurs regularly in nursing practice, even if nurses don't consider themselves "innovators" as such. Consider how often nurses change systems so their work is easier to perform and so patient outcomes improve! The fact is, nurses innovate their way through every shift; we just call their innovations "workarounds." We must leverage that spirit of innovation to resolve our current nursing and healthcare crisis.

Nurse Innovators

Nurses might not think of themselves as innovators, but they are. For proof, one need look no further than the positive deviance among nurses, the workarounds they devise, and their critical-thinking skills.

Nurses have *always* been innovators. Indeed, innovation is an intrinsic part of healthcare, as every new patient presents their own host of problems to solve. Nursing innovations have included hand hygiene, the crash cart, the feeding tube, and the use of sunlight to resolve the jaundice of newborns, to name just a few.

In recent years, thousands of nurses have become leaders in innovation. Some have even built multimillion dollar companies, including companies offering a system of Federally Qualified Health Centers, nursing scheduling platforms, nurse social connection apps, nursing licensure certification, portfolio manager platforms, concierge nursing models, virtual nursing technologies—the list goes on.

These nurse innovators often go unnoticed. This is perhaps because nurses are typically humble and quiet. Even our own colleagues may be unaware of our amazing work and the impact we make. We should rethink this. We should celebrate these achievements, loudly and openly. Nurses are successful innovators and entrepreneurs, and we don't talk about that enough.

"

"Nurses think of innovation as a one off or 'extra' versus embracing the process such as the regular workarounds or MacGyvering that they do shift after shift just to care for patients. Innovation is the backdrop to frame the influence of nurses and harness the power of the profession."

–Dr. Jeff Adams

"

TRANSFORMATION

Transformation describes "profound, fundamental change, altering the very nature of something," says Gass. Moreover, "Transformational change is both radical and sustainable. Something that is transformed can never go back to exactly what it was before" (Gass, 2012, para. 1).

Transforming systems through innovation is as much about developing new models of care, new practices, and new processes as it is about developing new technologies, new devices, or new applications (apps). Transformation can even involve social innovation to reduce or eliminate disparities, improve health equity, or reduce the impact of social determinants of health by tackling big social challenges such as food insecurity or homelessness.

Transformation through innovation requires inputs, feedback, and data, which may be hard to obtain. Furthermore, decision-making to advance innovation must continue even in the absence of precise or real-time data. Fortunately, our critical-thinking skills can help us make safe decisions based on what we know at the time. We nurses do this all the time, deciding to the best of our ability whether to progress or cease forward movement by using our expertise, training, developed skills, and competence and collaborating with our cross-functional team.

COMPLEX ADAPTIVE SYSTEMS

A *complex adaptive system (CAS)* generally involves biology, mathematics, complexity science, and physics. Essentially, a CAS is where human behavior and complexity science meet. An important characteristic of a CAS is that it must be dynamic enough to adapt to a rapidly changing environment. A complex adaptive system represents "a densely linked, intersecting, and interacting connection of agents, each making their own contribution and acting both independently in making that contribution and interdependently in linking that contribution to the independent but related contributions of other agents" (Weberg & Mangold, 2023, p. 355). Essentially, this defines the current state of healthcare.

VUCA

The acronym VUCA—which stands for *volatile, uncertain, complex, ambiguous*—has been around since 1987 (Mindtools, n.d.). It became popular among the military and intelligence community after the 9/11 attacks to describe the theater of battle and to help leaders think through planning scenarios. However, the term is also an appropriate frame of reference for our healthcare ecosystem. Indeed, the words *volatile, uncertain, complex,* and *ambiguous* effectively define our current healthcare environment:

- **Volatile:** It often feels as though unpredictable changes and/or transitions could occur within the healthcare ecosystem with short or no notice at any time.

- **Uncertain:** There is a lack of clarity regarding our healthcare ecosystem at the present time, and there is uncertainty about the future.

- **Complex:** There are multiple confusing and potentially chaotic factors in each healthcare scenario/equation.

- **Ambiguous:** There is little evidence of situational awareness and/or clarity within our healthcare ecosystem.

As a result, what we used to be able to somewhat predict, we can no longer even come close to predicting, and what we used to be able to see coming is now upon us before we know what to do. And while it's true that data analytics can help our mortal brains catch up, our models are only as good as our assumptions.

Our VUCA world has a powerful impact on organizations, ecosystems, and team members, and it can have an overall destabilizing effect. While some people and organizations thrive on uncertainty and pressure, others struggle with it. Leaders who evolve and continually build new networks and systems can create organizations that thrive in a VUCA environment. One way to achieve this is to evaluate strategic plans through a VUCA filter. This enables us to acknowledge the difficulties of the current and foreseeable future, identify things that may go wrong, and plan accordingly.

KNOWNS AND UNKNOWNS

Understanding the difficulties of operating within the current healthcare environment requires an understanding of *knowns*, *unknowns*, and *unknown-unknowns*—a concept identified by Secretary of State Donald Rumsfeld after 9/11 (Atkinson, 2020).

Although incorporating what you know and what you don't know into a planning process is by no means easy, it is worth the effort, particularly for organizations that are working to transform. Understanding the dynamic nature of the environment that we are in—and considering in advance that it is only going to become even more complex—provides a framework for long-term solutions. A Johari window (see Figure 2.1) provides an organized way to think about knowns and unknowns.

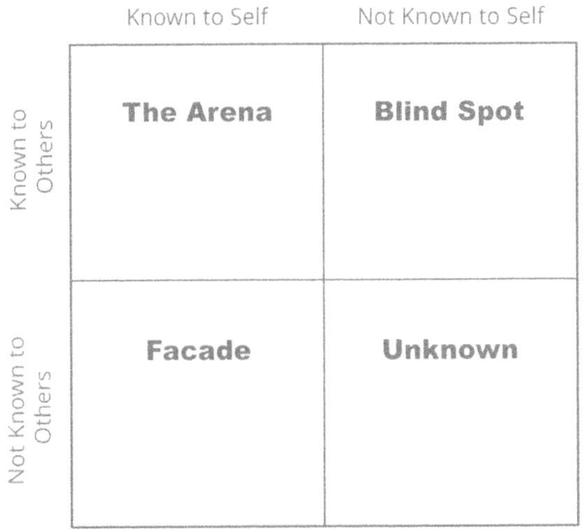

	Known to Self	Not Known to Self
Known to Others	**The Arena**	**Blind Spot**
Not Known to Others	**Facade**	**Unknown**

Figure 2.1 Johari window (Johari window, 2022).

RESILIENCE

Resilience is defined as "the capability of a strained body to recover its size and shape after deformation caused especially by compressive stress" or as an "ability to recover from or adjust to misfortune or change" (Merriam-Webster, n.d.).

Many modern nurses hold a certain amount of contempt for resilience, likely because this overused term seems to imply a certain level of individual weakness. However, resilience is an important concept as we learn how to support nurses and nurse leaders through an extremely difficult period of time. In this context, *resilience* should refer to the ongoing process of helping staff and leaders manage stress and cope with a dynamic health-care ecosystem.

Resilience is like a muscle. It needs training. Both nurses and leaders should train to manage the stresses associated with their work, just like professional athletes train to perform at their peak. This training should start in nursing school and continue on a regular basis to protect and sustain our profession.

"If you look at history, innovation doesn't come just from giving people incentives; it comes from creating environments where their ideas can connect."

–Steven Johnson

CONCLUSION

Transforming the current healthcare environment requires thoughtful and creative navigation, willingness to disrupt every facet, and a plethora of new tools, not to mention recognizing the need for change and embracing the hard work needed to effect it. But first, it means understanding the nomenclature around transformation.

Diversity of thought and novel approaches to nurse-led innovation will guide the future of care-delivery models. Nurses are notoriously good at thinking on their feet and solving problems in real-time. As leaders attempting to transform healthcare despite its VUCA nature, we must gratefully acknowledge the role of the positive deviant and apply the term "how might we" to every challenge. And of course, we must keep our nurses' resilience in mind as we look for ways to relieve the friction associated with care delivery. This alone will be a welcome change!

REFERENCES

Atkinson, P. (2020, September 5). *Unknown unknowns: Managing change post pandemic.* http://www.philipatkinson.com/blogculturechange/unknown-unknowns-managing-change-post-pandemic

Bestsennyy, O., Chmielewski, M., Koffel, A., & Shah, A. (2022, February 1). *From facility to home: How healthcare could shift by 2025.* https://www.mckinsey.com/industries/healthcare-systems-and-services/our-insights/from-facility-to-home-how-healthcare-could-shift-by-2025

Gary, J. C. (2013). Exploring the concept and use of positive deviance in nursing. *American Journal of Nursing, 113* (8), 26–34.

Gass, R. (2012). *What is transformation?* https://strategiesforsocialchange.com/wp-content/uploads/2016/01/what_is_transformation_2.0_lowrres.pdf

Johari window. (2022, November 29). In *Wikipedia.* https://en.wikipedia.org/wiki/File:Johari_Window.PNG

Johnson & Johnson. (2018, November 12). *Nurse innovator & entrepreneur emphasizes adding value to patient care.* https://nursing.jnj.com/nurse-innovator-entrepreneur-emphasizes-adding-value-to-patient-care?fbclid=IwAR1n9iI0mR_ByoC6sSZfMZOfDwgRYUaCqrlJjqcwb-UOu9_ehVIM0kPiRa0

Mate, K. (2017, March 23). *What's the difference between innovation and improvement?* Institute for Healthcare Improvement. https://www.ihi.org/communities/blogs/_layouts/15/ihi/community/blog/itemview.aspx?List=7d1126ec-8f63-4a3b-9926-c44ea3036813&ID=375#:~:text=The%20mental%20model%20in%20improvement,be%20further%20optimized%20using%20improvement

Melnyk, B. M., & Davidson, S. (2009, October–December). Creating a culture of innovation in nursing education through shared vision, leadership, interdisciplinary partnerships, and positive deviance. *Nursing Administration Quarterly, 33*(4), 288–295.

Merriam–Webster. (n.d.). Resilience. In *Merriam–Webster.com dictionary*. Retrieved September 5, 2022, from https://www.merriam-webster.com/dictionary/resilience

Mindtools. (n.d.). *Managing in a VUCA world*. https://www.mindtools.com/pages/article/managing-vuca-world.htm#:~:text=VUCA%20stands%20for%20volatility%2C%20uncertaintyday%2Dto%2Dday%20working

Murphy, Bill Jr. (2020, November 1). *Google says it still uses the '20 percent rule,' and you should totally copy it*. Inc. https://www.inc.com/bill-murphy-jr/google-says-it-still-uses-20-percent-rule-you-should-totally-copy-it.html

Petrie, D. A., & Swanson, R. C. (2018). The mental demands of leadership in complex adaptive systems. *Healthcare Management Forum, 31*(5), 206–213.

Thakur, R., Hsu, S. H. Y., & Fontenot, G. (2012). Innovation in healthcare: Issues and future trends. *Journal of Business Research, 65*(4), 562–569.

Weberg, D., & Davidson, S. (2021). *Leadership for evidence-based innovation in nursing and health professions* (2nd ed.). Jones & Bartlett Learning.

Weberg, D., & Mangold, K. (2023). *Leadership in nursing practice: The intersection of innovation and teamwork in healthcare systems* (4th ed.). Jones & Bartlett Learning.

"Culture eats strategy for breakfast."

—Peter Drucker

CHAPTER 3

Culture as the Foundation of Innovation

KEYWORDS

Change management, culture, culture transformation, healthy work environment, influence, diffusion of innovation, entrepreneur, intrapreneur

This chapter highlights concepts and tools—like Schein's model of organizational culture, the Adams influence model (AIM), and Kotter's 8-step change model—that relate to the importance of a positive work environment, strong workplace culture, and capitalizing on influence. These concepts and tools will help you create a culture in which innovation can thrive.

OBJECTIVES

- Explain the importance of culture in transformation work.
- Describe key characteristics associated with building a culture of innovation.

We started this chapter with a famous quote from management consultant Peter Drucker: "Culture eats strategy for breakfast." This quote does not imply that strategy is less important than culture; rather, it means that nothing can be accomplished if the culture does not permit it.

Although a negative workplace culture and environment are not the only problems we have in nursing, they are among the most fixable. This is why every organization should be focused on building a positive culture: to provide the foundation needed for every *other* initiative. If we don't create positive, supportive, safe, and respectful workplaces, we cannot fix the churn that we are currently experiencing in nursing.

CULTURE IS EVERYTHING

Let's face it: Workplace culture remains a problem in nursing. It's no secret that nurses must deal with pettiness, cliques, favoritism, incivility, and bullying from coworkers, other members of the care team, and patients and their families. This isn't new; negative behaviors like these have been a problem for as long as nursing has existed as a profession. And of course, the COVID-19 pandemic has exacerbated this behavior.

Creating a positive work environment—and with it a cohesive, desirable workplace culture—is a necessary step in building a profession that attracts and retains the best and the brightest. But a positive work environment isn't just one with positivity and hugs. Rather, it's one that supports those who experience moral injury, burnout, and the ongoing trauma associated with caregiving.

A positive work environment is essential. If you have ever been employed someplace where the work was tough and the hours ground you down, but the people you worked with kept you going, then you understand what the end goal is. Being supported and *knowing* the value your peers place on you and your work is one of the best feelings in the world. Not everyone has the opportunity to experience this; I have only twice.

---

ff

"Culture and the way people treat each other are more important than pay, benefits, and schedules. Recent studies have shown that an underlying cause of burnout and turnover is bullying and incivility. It is the healthcare organizations that have the responsibility to support and equip their leaders with the skills and tools they need to finally start addressing disruptive behaviors."

–Dr. Renee Thompson

JJ

FOSTERING A POSITIVE CULTURE

Creating and maintaining a positive culture is among the hardest work that leaders do. It's particularly challenging mostly because it involves uniting people who have their own opinions, styles, and goals and who play different roles. Some are nurses, some are other types of healthcare professionals, and some are unlicensed personnel, each with different training and values. They also have generational, cultural, and communication differences, not to mention different belief systems. And of course, they work in a complex, dynamic, and high-stress environment. So, although the diversity of thought that characterizes the staff in any healthcare organization makes us stronger, it also complicates the process of creating a work environment that everyone wants to be a part of.

Fostering a positive environment requires a steady supply of positivity. Typically, this positive energy emanates from the organizational leaders and from team members who want to make a positive contribution. Unfortunately, most organizations also employ plenty of people whose energy is negative or even toxic. These people suck the joy, camaraderie, and upbeat attitudes from those around them. They create a cycle of stress and angst by sowing doubts, talking about people instead of problems, pitting staff against each other, and pushing the limits of agreed-upon norms.

Once negative behaviors have been observed or reported, management must deal with toxic staff members appropriately, as quickly as possible. Leaders must intervene to address negative behavior by stopping the source of the toxicity and/or creating a positive support network to offset it (Weberg & Davidson, 2021). Sometimes, leaders contribute to a negative environment by deciding that it's less trouble to leave a negative element in place than to deal with it properly—an attitude of "The devil you know is better than the devil you don't." Particularly since the onset of the COVID-19 pandemic, it is common for leaders experiencing significant staffing shortages to decide that having a "warm body" is better than being short-staffed, and they will therefore accept negative behavior and poor performance. In the long run, this is a great way to lose all of the middle- and high-performing staff and find yourself with only poor performers.

> Deal with toxic staff swiftly and appropriately. Remember, what you permit you promote. Other staff will take notice.

"

"Culture does not change because we desire to change it. Culture changes when the organization is transformed—the culture reflects the realities of people working together every day."

–Frances Hesselbein

"

SCHEIN'S MODEL OF ORGANIZATIONAL CULTURE

Whether a culture is positive or negative, welcoming or isolating, it sets the tone for how employees feel as they perform their job—which in turn affects how patients, families, and visitors feel they are cared for and treated.

Schein's model of organizational culture identifies three main components of organizational culture:

- Norms of communication

- How people act

- Organizational artifacts, such as the posters in a department or photos on the lobby walls (Schein, 2010)

You can use Schein's model to build a positive culture—mitigating the negative elements you can't change and fixing the ones that you can. For example, you could change the norms of communication for shift reports by moving them to the bedside.

In addition to being more collegial, this makes managing each other up part of the report process. It might feel fake or contrived at first, but as staff warm to the idea, and if they respect and even like their peers, an authentic conversation—one of mutual respect—will develop during the bedside report.

One way to change how people act is to ensure you hear from all voices during staff meetings by intentionally pulling in the quiet, satisfied staff to balance out the loud, dissatisfied staff, who often share more openly and broadly. Also insist on mutual respect as well as tolerance for differing opinions to demonstrate the importance of hearing from everyone. And of course, guide the team using positive thoughts, ideas, and solutions.

On the subject of organizational artifacts, hospitals tend to display way too many signs, notices, and alerts—so many, in fact, that after a while, employees become completely oblivious to them. This might sound silly, but eliminating signage clutter has a subliminal positive impact on people's mood and behavior, the same way cleaning up a cluttered room does. You can then replace some of the clutter with quotes and images—for example, photos of a staff member's new baby or pet photos. Simply changing the organizational artifacts can create a more positive and welcoming culture.

CREATING A SAFE WORK ENVIRONMENT

Many healthcare workplaces are negative and toxic, which has a serious effect on nurses' mental health, wellbeing, burnout, and turnover. A 2022 survey with 11,863 nurse respondents showed that 60% of nurses have experienced "violence, bullying or incivility" at work—42% from fellow staff members (American Nurses Foundation, 2022).

This is completely unacceptable. No one should *ever* have to put up with this sort of behavior. Nursing is long overdue for a tough stand against incivility. We absolutely must adopt a profession-wide, zero-tolerance policy regarding incivility—a standard that is set and enforced by licensing, regulation, and accrediting bodies, akin to the American Nurses Association's Racial Reckoning Statement against racism in nursing (American Nurses Association, 2022). No matter how skilled or experienced a nurse is, if they are uncivil, they must go. This is why our culture work is so important now. It's a necessary step in creating practice environments in which people actually want to work, not to mention the impact it will have on retention—not just of nurses, but of everyone else in the organization, too. (Turnover doesn't only affect nurses!)

Perhaps even more concerning than the 42% of nurses who have experienced violence, bullying, or incivility at the hands of their colleagues are the 55% who have experienced it with patients, and the 49% who've experienced it with patients' families. Zero tolerance of abuse and violence goes for patients and their visitors, too. Several hospitals have begun placing signage to this effect at all entrances, but we need more. It is time for the passage of a nationwide law that holds patients and family members accountable, similar to the Protection from Abusive Passengers Act, which federal lawmakers passed in April 2022 to protect airline pilots and flight crews (Congress.gov, 2022).

Of course, the underpinnings of violence are complex behavioral health issues that often require mental health treatment.

BUILDING A CULTURE OF INNOVATION

With a supportive and healthy work environment in place, the real work of transformation can begin. For innovation to thrive within an organization, leaders must exhibit five salient characteristics (Cianelli et al., 2016):

- **Divergent thinking:** This involves the ability of an organization to think broadly and creatively. It means *not* zeroing in on solutions with a preconceived notion, but rather, being open to all possibilities. Often called *blue-sky thinking,* divergent thinking is very open-minded. It's the opposite of *convergent thinking,* which is more linear and laser-focused on a solution.

- **Risk-taking:** In healthcare, *risk-taking* refers to calculated and considered risks that keep patient safety and the safety of the healthcare team as a primary concern. In healthcare, there are often processes and systems that could be changed, but we just aren't always open to doing things in new ways. In fact, there is a common saying in healthcare that I think encapsulates this attitude: "*That* isn't how we do it here." This kind of risk-averse, closed-minded thinking has created many of the current challenges in nursing and in healthcare overall. When evaluating new programs, devices, and processes, be thoughtful. And where appropriate, step out of your comfort zone to take a calculated and well-considered risk.

- **Failure tolerance:** The saying "fail fast and fail often" sounds frightening. But it really just refers to the fact that early stumbles in a pilot or change-management process are good learning opportunities and can help you create an even stronger foundation for success. Think about the failures that so many people have experienced before becoming successful. A great example is Thomas Edison! He experimented with thousands of light bulbs before finding success. Learning from failure is important to your eventual success when transforming a system.

- **Agility and flexibility:** The ability of an organization to quickly adapt to rapidly changing trends is not only important, but necessary for an organization's survival. *Agility* is the "capability to adjust swiftly in response to market changes" (Cianelli et al., 2016, p. 9). In contrast, *flexibility* is the ability to "provide different outcomes with the same resources by expanding, contracting and redistributing resources to meet emerging needs" (Cianelli et al., 2016, p. 9). Organizations that are agile and flexible are often described as *nimble*. Being nimble is something we must strive for.

- **Autonomy and freedom:** Providing leaders and employees the latitude to do what they do best is often said but rarely done. Simply put, creating an organizational ecosystem in which everyone is free to problem-solve and share their ideas is the exception, not the norm. Too many organizations are full of people who keep their heads down, do what they are told, and go home at the end of their shift. These are not the conditions for innovation. Innovative organizations are places where everyone contributes, shares, and provides constructive feedback to make the organization better. But be aware that it's not enough to simply encourage all members of your team to contribute to the organization's greater goals. You must also empower them by ensuring they have adequate time and resources to do so. In addition, you must do more than ask for feedback; you must actually listen to that feedback and act on it.

> The most innovative organizations strongly encourage ideas and feedback from all levels of staff—and communicate robustly regarding the outcomes.

DIFFUSING INNOVATION THROUGHOUT AN ORGANIZATION

Change doesn't just happen. There's often a process to how a new idea gains traction and spreads through a population, such as a department or organization.

The diffusion of innovation theory by Everett Rogers helps us to understand this process. The term *diffusion* refers to the adoption of the new idea or innovation. According to Rogers, for adoption to occur, people need to "perceive the idea, behavior or product as new or innovative" (Boston University School of Public Health, 2022, para. 1).

The diffusion of innovation theory also suggests that different people adopt new ideas or innovations at different rates. Rogers divides these people, or adopters, into five categories, each with its own traits and characteristics. Rogers also identifies different strategies that can be used to engage members of each category to adopt a new idea or innovation. These categories are as follows:

- **Innovators:** These are people who like new things and want to be the first to try an innovation. They are often described as curious, creative, and risk-takers. Not much effort is required to convince an innovator to try or do something new, as they are eager to implement change (Boston University School of Public Health, 2022, para. 2).

- **Early adopters:** This cohort might not be as enthusiastic as innovators, but they are ready and willing to adopt something new. They are often leaders and look for opportunities to change. This group only needs to be pointed in a new direction and given a how-to; from there, they will manage the change themselves (Boston University School of Public Health, 2022, para. 2).

- **Early majority:** Members of this group are not seen as leaders, even though they may adopt new ideas before the average person. Sharing "evidence of effectiveness" and personal success stories is a good way to motivate this group to change (Boston University School of Public Health, 2022, para. 2).

- **Late majority:** This cohort is very skeptical of any new idea or behavior and will only adopt it after the majority has already done so. You can move this group toward progress by sharing with them who has already adopted the change and what their experience has been (Boston University School of Public Health, 2022, para. 2).

- **Laggards:** This group is often described as conservative. They are generally unwilling to try new things. It is very difficult to motivate this group to try or do something new. They might require much convincing, including frequent sharing of data and pressure from others who have already adopted the new idea or behavior (Boston University School of Public Health, 2022, para. 2).

Figure 3.1 shows a typical breakdown of these categories. It is likely that members of your own organization will follow the same adoption curve. Consider where you fit in this model and how you might help those who may be behind you.

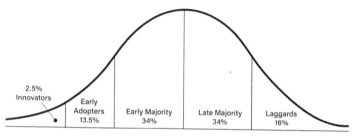

FIGURE 3.1 Diffusion of innovation.

ENTREPRENEURS AND INTRAPRENEURS

A good way to promote organizational innovation is to cultivate a cadre of entrepreneurs and intrapreneurs. An *entrepreneur* is "one who organizes, manages and assumes the risks of a business or enterprise" (Merriam-Webster, n.d., para. 1). Another way to think about entrepreneurs is "a person who organizes and manages any enterprise, especially a business, usually with considerable initiative and risk" (Dictionary.com, n.d., para. 1). In contrast, an *intrapreneur* is someone who innovates and generates new ideas within an organization with a goal of driving change. If you constantly come up with new ideas at work, you are an intrapreneur!

Intrapreneurship is very similar to entrepreneurship in that it drives positive change, but it does so without the risk involved in leaving the organization (Clipper et al., 2019). And intrapreneurs typically exhibit the same characteristics and traits as those associated with entrepreneurs, such as creativity, curiosity, resilience, a passion for learning, and the ability to tolerate failure.

Creating the conditions for intrapreneurs to flourish fosters engagement, promotes innovation, and can produce exciting results. It also unleashes and empowers those closest to the work to go forth and innovate. Imagine the impact of an army of small-business owners operating as problem-solvers and change agents in the healthcare arena. That is the benefit of deploying intrapreneurs within your organization!

> Innovating out of the current chaos in healthcare to create a sustainable future for nursing will require both entrepreneurs and intrapreneurs.

> " *"If your actions create a legacy that inspires others to dream more, learn more, do more and become more, then, you are an excellent leader."*
>
> –Dolly Parton

THE IMPACT OF LEADERSHIP

Leaders often play the most influential role in innovation and transformation, acting as support systems, educators, catalysts, and change champions. But in today's chaotic environment, leadership is an extreme sport. The result is that, in addition to the increase in turnover of direct care nurses, there is also an increase in turnover of nursing leaders, including managers, directors, and chief nurse executives. In fact, in a 2021 study of nearly 2,000 nursing leaders across 47 states, over 50% of them indicated that they intended to leave their current positions within the next five years (Warden et al., 2021). Breaking down these numbers, among nurse managers, the percentage was 51.4%; among nurse directors, the percentage was 49.6%; and among nurse executives, the percentage was 52.9% (Warden et al., 2021, p. 878).

The rationale for leaving differed from role to role. For nurse executives, retirement was the top reason. For nurse directors, retirement tied with advancement in a different organization as the top cause. And for nurse managers, burnout was the number one driver (Warden et al., 2021, p. 880). This is not surprising, because nurse managers are caught between leadership and staff—they are often responsible for the same work as the regular staff but are expected to perform leadership duties too. In any case, whenever a nurse leader exits an organization, it takes months to fill the vacant position—and even longer to bring the new (or interim) person up to speed so they can function effectively as a leader. It goes without saying that this process also has a negative impact on the team.

Of course, the role of the nurse leader has always been personally taxing and seemed never-ending. But in today's environment, the job of a nurse leader is literally 24/7/365. It is virtually impossible to succeed. This situation requires an immediate call to action. If we want to identify new care models, we must first reverse these turnover trends. This means ensuring our nursing leaders feel valued, appreciated, and successful. Otherwise, we risk even higher rates of leader turnover, and other key staff will likely follow them out the door. Addressing the issues that nursing leaders say drive them out of the profession is crucial.

There's not much we can do to affect retirement age. But we *can* minimize burnout by making the role of a nurse executive more doable and by helping them be successful. After all, it is in everyone's best interest if leaders succeed! In doing so, we may be able to persuade older nurses to lend us their skills and organizational knowledge for a few more years.

This requires change at both the system level (unit, department, organization) *and* the individual level, resulting in a symbiotic partnership that supports an ecosystem of success.

One possible solution is to pilot and test job-sharing programs for managers, directors, and even chief nurse executives. This was a popular approach in the late 1970s and early 1980s, but it fell to the wayside because accommodating the growing numbers of nurse leaders became less important to healthcare organizations than initiatives to improve efficiency and cut costs. Another possible solution is to explore work-from-home options; as we discovered during the COVID-19 pandemic, there is an appetite for this model. While working from home is difficult (or impossible) in many areas of healthcare, it could work for nurse leaders who don't provide direct patient care, even if only in a limited way. A third possible solution is to adjust expectations of nurse leader work schedules. For example, instead of five days a week, for eight hours a day (which, let's face it, often becomes six or seven days a week, for 10 to 12 hours a day), leaders could work three or four days a week, for 10 or 12 hours a day. Or nurse leaders could work from home one day each week (as long as there is sufficient staffing onsite). Finally, we could try tapping retired leaders to mentor up-and-coming ones to make them more effective and successful. Ultimately, there are no clear or easy answers here. But this moment represents an opportunity for a reset. We have a mandate to get creative, automate what we can, set realistic performance expectations, and collaborate directly with leaders to redesign their roles.

For leaders, building a culture of innovation requires focus and effort. Beyond that, leaders should also serve as mentors and role models for innovation. Nurse leaders play a particularly large part in empowering their teams to generate ideas and solutions and in providing them with the necessary resources to do so. They can also assist in advancing these ideas and solutions through the prescribed organizational channels for evaluation and perhaps further development. To achieve this, innovation should be a regular topic of discussion—for example, during departmental leader rounding and during meetings. Whether the solutions that bubble up from staff succeed or not, the goal is to create a culture where ideas *can* flourish given the right support and resources, and to recognize and celebrate innovation when it occurs. While many organizations funnel this work through innovation-based resources, others use their existing performance-improvement resources to evaluate and advance solutions.

Sometimes innovation is disruptive and transformative. Other times, though, ideas and solutions from staff are more incremental in nature. Still, your organization should welcome this type of innovation.

To be successful, innovation and transformation may require a change in management, depending on how agile the organization is. This can be true of disruptive innovation as well as incremental innovation.

Leading Innovation

Weberg and Mangold (2023, p. 55) have identified leadership traits that increase the likelihood of success in innovation and transformation. These traits are:

- Self-aware
- Courageous and hopeful
- Proactive and future-oriented
- Inquisitive and optimistic
- Able to experiment and remediate

LEVERAGING CHANGE MANAGEMENT PRACTICES

Innovative ideas and solutions without successful execution and adoption won't accomplish much. But successful execution and adoption are difficult. Complicating matters, it's often the case that several changes are happening at once, making it difficult for staff to prioritize what they often think of as the "initiative of the month."

One way for leaders to ensure that changes are deployed across an organization at the right time and in the right order, and to improve the chances that the changes will stick, is to leverage change-management practices. Change management is an important leadership competency to master. However, change management can be difficult—which is why more than 70% of organizational changes fail (Jain, 2019).

To increase the chances of success, it helps to adopt an organizational change model or framework and to use it for any and all changes rolled out, no matter who owns the change. One simple, common-sense, and effective change model is Kotter's 8-step change model (Kotter, n.d.). This model spells out eight necessary steps to create long-lasting change within an organization. (See Figure 3.2.) In addition to assisting in hard-wiring organizational level change, this model can also be applied to smaller settings, such as units, departments, or even specific shifts.

> The change model that an organization uses should be clearly communicated during orientation, as it is as important as the mission, vision, and values.

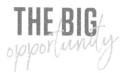

CREATE
A SENSE OF URGENCY

INSTITUTE
CHANGE

BUILD
A GUIDING COALITION

SUSTAIN
ACCELERATION

THE BIG opportunity

FORM
A STRATEGIC VISION

GENERATE
SHORT-TERM WINS

ENABLE
ACTION BY REMOVING BARRIERS

ENLIST
A VOLUNTEER ARMY

FIGURE 3.2 Kotter's 8-step change model (Kotter, n.d.). Used with permission.

Step 1: Create a Sense of Urgency

When starting a change initiative, it is incredibly important to create a sense of urgency. This includes explaining the reason for the change and why it must be done at this time (Kotter, 2007). To effectively lead the change initiative, it is also important to solicit the buy-in of at least 75% of the organizational leadership team (Jain, 2019).

Step 2: Form a Guiding Coalition

Forming a guiding coalition of leadership champions and key stakeholders—which should include leaders from different levels as well as diversity of thought—is crucial (Kotter, 2007).

Step 3: Create a Strategic Vision

Change can be stressful and difficult to understand. So, it is important to communicate a vision of where the organization is headed and what success will look like (Kotter, 2007). The more clearly this can be documented, and the more frequently and consistently it can be shared, the more likely it is that members of the organization will understand the organization's vision. Paint the picture of the future state.

Step 4: Initiate Change Communication

There are lots of logistics associated with change management, but the most important ones are messaging and communicating change (Kotter, 2007). The clearer and more frequent the communication is, the more likely it will be received. A good rule of thumb is to communicate seven times, in seven ways. That is, communicate the vision and the reason for the change frequently and through different modalities—for example, town hall meetings, daily huddles, posters in break rooms, table tents in the cafeteria, the organizational intranet site, employee apps, emails to staff, and a variety of other means. The important thing is that this communication must occur consistently over and over again so the organization understands the change and how it is progressing.

Step 5: Remove Barriers to Change

Organizational change initiatives are often met with resistance. In fact, organizational friction is a common response to change. The leadership team must identify potential sources of friction or barriers in advance, and it must plan to mitigate them (Kotter, 2007). If the leaders themselves are the barriers, this should be gently brought to light through private conversations to build support for the change initiative. Because barriers can be dynamic throughout the change process, continue to evaluate any issues you encounter and your responses to those issues for the change initiative to be successful (Jain, 2019). Change is hard.

Step 6: Generate Short-Term Wins

Implementing change that sticks is a long and tedious process. It is not uncommon for the leadership team to move on to the next challenge before they complete the previous one (Kotter, 2007). To motivate the organization to maintain the change, find ways to recognize individuals, teams, and departments for their efforts, their contributions to the change initiative, and their success in the change process (Jain, 2019).

Step 7: Make Change a Continual Process

One way to ensure that change sticks is to develop SMART goals (Specific, Measurable, Achievable, Relevant, and Time-Bound) around the change, keep an eye on the outcomes, and analyze the effect of the change. Any change an organization measures and reports on will occur more quickly and stick for longer (Kotter, 2007).

Step 8: Incorporate Changes in the Organizational Culture

With any organizational change initiative, the expectation is that individuals within the organization make individual behavior changes to positively affect the overall outcome (Kotter, 2007). Ultimately, however, these changes must be hardwired. So, it's important to ensure that employees continually receive messaging and training around the change. Even organizational artifacts such as policies and procedures should reflect the change so it becomes woven into the fabric of the organization.

MASTERING INFLUENCE

In addition to mastering change management, nurse leaders must master the use of influence. In fact, to effect change, you must lean into influence hard. Influence is so important, the American Organization for Nursing Leadership (AONL) has codified the behaviors that facilitate it. These behaviors include:

- Asserting views in nonthreatening, nonjudgmental ways

- Creating a shared vision

- Facilitating consensus-building

- Inspiring desired behaviors and managing undesired behaviors

- Achieving outcomes through engaging stakeholders

- Promoting decisions that are patient-centered

- Applying situational leadership skills (American Organization for Nursing Leadership, 2015, p. 4)

To assist leaders with utilizing and amplifying influence, the Adams influence model (AIM) provides a "framework for understanding the factors, attributes and processes of influence" (Adams & Erickson, 2011, p. 186; see Figure 3.3.) Adams suggests that influence is interpersonal. An *influence agent* (the person who is trying to influence someone else) can use a variety of tactics to compel an *influence target* (the person the influence agent seeks to influence) to change their way of thinking. These tactics include sharing data and information, building coalitions, using persuasion, and potentially even collaborating with the target. These can be used individually or combined as needed. Meanwhile, there are various factors of influence, including levels of authority, communication traits, competence, status, time, and timing (Adams & Erickson, 2011, p. 187). Finally, the AIM acknowledges the ecosystem by indicating that influence is affected by personal, interpersonal, and even social systems. At various times during the influence process, the influence agent may tap into these systems to achieve the desired result (Adams & Erickson, 2011, p. 187).

> The AIM can be leveraged to influence change within an organization and across nursing—and to assist in the transformation of nursing as a whole.

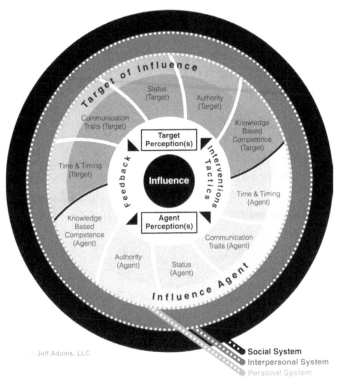

FIGURE 3.3   Adams influence model (Adams & Erickson, 2011). Used with permission.

USING OUR STATUS

Nursing has been voted "America's Most Trusted Profession" for 20 years in a row (Senior, 2022). This is an amazing honor, but it hasn't helped us advance our cause or reimagine nursing! It should, though.

As nurses, we often struggle to find our voice—or at least, a common and aligned voice. We often decry the healthcare industry's myopic focus on finances and productivity, but we have done little to change the system or even to advocate for policy change to address this.

If we nurses want change, then it's up to us to mobilize our collective voices—all 4.3 million of us—to drive it. Otherwise, if we allow the state of our profession to continue on its current path, we run the risk of being on the receiving end of change to our profession instead of driving the changes within our profession. We must use our influence to create a path through all the noise.

CONCLUSION

This chapter ends where it started: highlighting the fact that without a positive, optimistic, supportive culture, transformation cannot succeed. The importance of creating a respectful, safe workplace cannot be overstated. It is essential in constructing a solid foundation from which innovation can flourish and transformation can take shape.

Explore the tools and concepts described in this chapter. Then, once you feel competent using them, share them among your colleagues and eventually your organization as a whole. These frameworks can help your innovation work succeed and spread throughout the entire organization.

Creating the changes necessary to positively affect nursing is difficult. Change is hard, innovation is harder, and transformation is the hardest of all. But by using tools in collaboration with others to help catalyze change, to manage change, and advance new processes, we *will* succeed!

REFERENCES

Adams, J. M., & Erickson, J. I. (2011). Applying the Adams influence model in nurse executive practice. *Journal of Nursing Administration, 41*(4), 186–92.

American Nurses Association. (2022). *Racial reckoning statement.* https://www.nursingworld.org/practice-policy/workforce/racism-in-nursing/RacialReckoningStatement/

American Nurses Foundation. (2022). *Pulse on the nation's nurses COVID-19 survey series: Workplace survey, June–July 2022.* https://www.nursingworld.org/practice-policy/work-environment/health-safety/disaster-preparedness/coronavirus/what-you-need-to-know/covid-19-survey-series-anf-2022-workplace-survey/

American Organization for Nursing Leadership. (2015). *AONE nurse executive competencies.* https://www.aonl.org/sites/default/files/aone/nec.pdf

Boston University School of Public Health. (2022). Diffusion of innovation theory. https://sphweb.bumc.bu.edu/otlt/mph-modules/sb/behavioralchangetheories/behavioralchangetheories4.html

Cianelli, R., Clipper, B., Freeman, R., Goldstein, J., & Wyatt, T. (2016, June). *The innovation road map: A guide for nurse leaders.* Innovation Works.

Clipper, B., Wang, M., Coyne, P., Baiera, V., Love, R., Nix, D., Nix, W., & Weirich, B. (2019). *The nurse's guide to innovation.* Superstar Press.

Congress.gov. (2022). *H.R.7433 – Protection from Abusive Passengers Act.* https://www.congress.gov/bill/117th-congress/house-bill/7433/text?r=55&s=1

Dictionary.com. (n.d.). *Entrepreneur.* Retrieved August 18, 2020, from https://www.dictionary.com/browse/entrepreneur

Jain, M. (2019, December 3). *How to apply Kotter's 8–step change model.* https://whatfix.com/blog/kotters-8-step-change-model/

Kotter. (n.d.). *The 8 steps for leading change.* https://www.kotterinc.com/methodology/8-steps/

Kotter, J. P. (2007). Leading change: Why transformation efforts fail. *Harvard Business Review,* 2–9. https://hbr.org/2007/01/leading-change-why-transformation-efforts-fail

Merriam–Webster. (n.d.). Entrepreneur. In *Merriam–Webster.com dictionary.* Retrieved August 18, 2020, from https://www.merriam-webster.com/dictionary/entrepreneurship?utm_campaign=sd&utm_medium=serp&utm_source=jsonld

Schein, E. H. (2010). *Organizational culture and leadership* (Vol. 2). John Wiley & Sons.

Senior, R. (2022, January 12). Numbers don't lie: Nursing most trusted profession again. *American Nurse Journal*. https://www.myamericannurse.com/numbers-dont-lie-nurses-most-trusted-again/

Warden, D. H., Hughes, R. G., Probst, J. C., Warden, D. N., & Adams, S. A. (2021, September–October). Current turnover intention among nurse managers, directors, and executives. *Nursing Outlook* 69(5), 875–885.

Weberg, D., & Davidson, S. (2021). *Leadership for evidence-based innovation in nursing and health professions* (2nd ed.). Jones & Bartlett Learning.

Weberg, D., & Mangold, K. (2023). *Leadership in nursing practice. The intersection of innovation and teamwork in healthcare systems* (4th ed.). Jones & Bartlett Learning.

CHAPTER 4

Leadership in Turbulent Times

KEYWORDS

Leadership competencies, strategic management, complexity leadership theory, succession planning, accountability

This chapter shares leadership concepts that bolster support and provides tools for leaders to navigate transformation in their organizations. It covers topics such as change management and change models and tactics to measure success and to bake in accountability. These help maintain the momentum needed to lead during a transformation, which is critical given the scope and rate of change that all transformations require.

OBJECTIVES

- Articulate strategies to hold leaders accountable for change.
- Identify tactics for succession planning to assemble a deep bench of aspiring leaders for future roles.

The current healthcare environment requires new competencies, frameworks, and tools. Nurse leaders must discard old models that no longer prove useful and experiment with new ways of leading if the profession is to thrive in the future.

LEADERSHIP COMPETENCIES

Too often, leaders enter and leave healthcare organizations as though there's a revolving door. Worse, as one leader leaves, out of sheer desperation, we tend to plug the hole with a new leader who is not ready or someone who has not been properly prepared for the role. We must do a better job preparing, educating, and assisting our new leaders.

The American Organization for Nursing Leadership (AONL) recently updated the core competencies for nurse leadership to reflect similarities among various levels of leaders. The six domains are now:

- Communication and Relationship Building

- Leadership

- Knowledge of the Healthcare Environment and Clinical Principles

- Professionalism

- Business Skills and Principles

- "Leader Within" (Hughes et al., 2022, p. 1)

While all of these domains of competency are essential for a successful leader, two seem most germane to innovation and transformation:

- **Communication and Relationship Building:** This domain encompasses effective communication, relationship management, and influencing behaviors.

- **Leadership:** This domain pertains to systems and complex adaptive thinking, change management, transformation, and innovation.

STRATEGIC MANAGEMENT

Beyond the AONL nurse leader core competencies, modern-day nurse leaders need new competencies to broaden their thinking and drive innovation. These include the following:

- Data and analytics

- Innovation tools

- Human-centered design

- Entrepreneurship

- Artificial intelligence

> Think about how powerful it would be to have leaders who have actually started a business or sold a solution. Talk about knowing how to problem-solve and overcome barriers!

Artificial Intelligence Competencies for Nurses and Healthcare Professionals

- Basic knowledge of AI and healthcare applications

- Social and ethical implications of AI

- AI-enhanced clinical encounters (decision support, care planning, etc.)

- Evidence-based practice (EBP) evaluation of AI-based tools (quality, accuracy, safety, contextual appropriateness, and biases of tools and data sets)

- Workflow analysis for AI-based tools (teams, roles, responsibilities, and workflows)
- Practice-based learning and improvement (teams, workflows/workload, etc; Russell et al., 2022)

COMPLEXITY LEADERSHIP THEORY

As we contemplate ways for leaders to be more successful in an ever-changing healthcare environment, it's important to consider complexity leadership theory (CLT). With CLT, the leader shifts from problem-solving to fostering an environment in which problems are solved through collaboration, accountability, and empowerment. CLT, which is dynamic in nature, focuses on collaboration, adaptation, and self-organization to attain innovative and transformative outcomes.

To achieve these outcomes, leaders exhibit three types of behaviors: enabling, administrative, and adaptive (Weberg & Davidson, 2021, p. 37). Unlike autocratic and controlling behaviors, these behaviors pave the way for interactions that create the conditions for the evolution of adaptive and innovative structures (Weberg & Davidson, 2021, p. 37). Leaders should not only develop an understanding of CLT but adopt this approach in today's VUCA healthcare world.

SUCCESSION PLANNING

In addition to building leadership competencies, nurse leaders must engage in succession planning in a more urgent and intentional manner. Hard-wired processes to assess every leader and aspiring leader should occur at a regular cadence. In addition, an annual performance evaluation should take place to ascertain whether a leader or aspiring leader seeks to move on (external) or move up (internal). For those looking to move on, there should be a succession plan in place, and for those looking to move up who have potential for promotion, there should be a structured, written plan to address their development needs. This type of discipline ensures the organization knows which leaders are preparing to leave and enables them to launch either a re-recruitment conversation or a search for a new leader in a timelier fashion to minimize disruption to the department.

> Having retired leaders mentor newer nurse leaders is a great way to prepare the next generation of nurse leaders and keep organizational knowledge circulating within the organization.

Lacking a strong pool from which to draw new leaders into your rotation as other leaders leave results in an unstable practice environment—one in which it is less desirable for nurses to work and in which patient care is inconsistent. Therefore, identifying staff members who may have potential to evolve into nurse leaders is crucial. A simple tool called the nine-box grid (see Figure 4.1), used in conjunction with or separate from the annual performance evaluation process (for example, six months after the annual evaluation is completed), can assist with this. Completing a nine-box grid for each aspiring leader can help you determine whether that person might develop into a successful leader with increasing scope and role in the organization (The nine-box grid for talent management, 2017).

> Using a talent-management/succession-planning tool like nine box requires the organization to invest time and money in adequate training, particularly as you go deeper into the organization to flesh out your leadership bench.

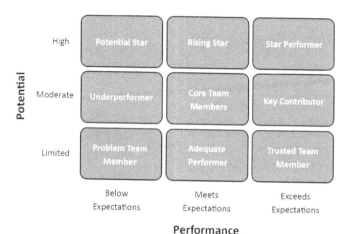

FIGURE 4.1   The nine-box grid for talent management (2017). Creative Commons.

REDESIGNING NURSE LEADERSHIP ROLES

Nurse leaders are rarely given the opportunity to participate in high-level organizational planning and strategy conversations. This is concerning. Nurses represent the largest cohort of labor in healthcare organizations. Moreover, nurses spend more time interacting with patients and their families than any other discipline. From now on, nurse leaders *must* be included in these planning and strategy sessions. This will require us to be more assertive and less apathetic. It might even mean we need to redesign our own roles. Nurse leaders must be at the table, and we need to get better at making a business case for change!

Redesigning the role of nurse leader also gives us a chance to make it more desirable and manageable. At present, nurse leaders often have a much broader span of control and responsibility than their non-nurse counterparts within the same organization. This is untenable. It's also one reason finding new nurse leaders keeps getting harder.

Redesigning leadership roles will require us to get very creative. We'll need to think completely outside the box. Otherwise, it will become increasingly difficult to recruit and retain nurse leaders.

> To successfully redesign leader roles, spend time with both current and aspiring leaders to identify needed changes.

One creative approach could be job-sharing manager and director roles, with two part-time leaders effectively functioning as one full-time leader. This would give each person downtime and time away; establish built-in boundaries around work hours and on-call expectations; and help both parties keep the job in perspective. Job-sharing was done successfully in the 1970s and 1980s, and it could work again in our current state. However, for job-sharing to be successful, there must be clear delineation of duties. In addition, organizations should provide both part-time leaders with full-time benefits. Remember, the goal is to recruit and retain the best leaders, not to save small dollar amounts on benefits.

Another creative solution is to tap non-nurses to complete non-nursing work currently performed by nurse leaders. For example, some organizations have successfully shifted time-intensive tasks like handling payroll and ordering supplies to support staff. Support staff or focused project managers could even monitor quality/practice improvement issues as well as maintain the cadence and milestones of important experience, quality, and safety initiatives within nursing departments or units. (Of course, both these solutions—and others—require the evaluation and possible revision of current nurse leader job descriptions.)

Some executives might resist adding new full-time employees (FTEs) or additional salaries. But doing so is well worth it. In addition to helping to keep goals and initiatives on track, a new approach will improve leader engagement and satisfaction.

> Steps like these do not diminish the importance of the nurse leader role; they simply make the job more doable.

Remember, leader recruitment and retention are the goals. Your only alternative is to continue experiencing high turnover among nurse leaders. Not only is this expensive, it affects patient safety and turnover of other staff.

A NEW TWIST ON CAREER MOBILITY

The current generation of new nurses wants faster career mobility, with shorter stays in any given role. To satisfy these nurses, organizations should consider creating career paths for entry-level nurses that encourage horizontal and vertical movement in shorter periods of time. Organizations that are uncomfortable about allowing shorter career paths for new nurses will need to become comfortable with it, or new nurses will find career opportunities elsewhere. The generational paradigm of career progression has shifted. It is not up to us to define it, but rather to adapt to it.

During orientation for new graduate nurses, make it a point to showcase successful clinical nurses and nurse leaders within the organization to inspire them and instill a vision for their own career trajectory. Then, develop a plan to help them achieve their own career goals on their timeline.

Some organizations offer meetings that could be compared to speed-dating sessions. In these, nurses who have been in the organization for less than one year interview more tenured nurses for five to eight minutes to hear about their experiences and gain career insights. This process reveals to less-tenured nurses what roles they could move into if they remain within the organization and what steps they might take to do so.

> Even if a new nurse decides to change departments, as long as they stay in your organization, it's a win-win.

Both of these approaches can prove effective in helping new nurses develop career paths. They can also instill in new nurses a sense of investment and loyalty. At the same time, they recognize the valuable contributions of their more experienced colleagues. All three of these outcomes are likely to promote retention within your organization.

Each generation thinks differently about their career path. For example, it's particularly important for Gen-Z nurses to imagine their future with an organization because generally speaking, they do not see themselves staying in any one place for more than two years. In fact, this is now the average amount of time a newly graduated nurse spends at the bedside before leaving for a new role (Advisory Board, 2021, slide 22). Millennials are holding steady or reducing hours based on life goals, Gen-X nurses are evaluating prospects for cutting back hours or perhaps even retiring, and baby boomer nurses are focused primarily on retirement.

As more tenured nurses and nurse leaders progress down their own career paths or retire from the profession, millennials and

Gen-Z nurses will shift into the majority of nursing and leadership roles. This shift will bring about significant change, which may help move us through our current challenges. As an example of a generational paradigm shift, we used to ask staff to cover up tattoos or wear long sleeves. Now tattoos are so commonplace in popular culture that we have had to adapt to accept tattoos. Otherwise, we wouldn't have enough staff!

BAKING IN ACCOUNTABILITY

Accountability is crucial to leadership success and in the achievement of organizational goals. Accountability requires three key characteristics (Weberg & Mangold, 2023):

- *Competence:* This is defined as the ability to safely, accurately, and/or correctly perform an action.

- *Autonomy:* This can be summed up as the ability to "make certain decisions or to take action" (Weberg & Mangold, 2023, p. 6).

- *Authority:* This is about having the power to make certain decisions or to determine or perform a certain action. Accountability without authority is meaningless.

Accountability also involves an investment in team members. Moreover, for it to be meaningful, accountability requires follow-up and consequences when appropriate. That is, there must be some process to ensure that the agreed-upon actions have actually been *done,* and if not, there must be repercussions. Otherwise, the result will be apathy and a lack of ownership, and nothing will change.

As an industry, healthcare would greatly benefit from more accountability. All too often, we are told that an initiative will be implemented, but at the end of the quarter, we are left to wonder if anything was actually accomplished. Execution almost always proves to be the hardest part of any strategy—particularly when there's no accountability.

Fortunately, there are models that provide a structured approach to establish accountability and provide shared clarity. The benefits of implementing these types of tools within a dynamic healthcare ecosystem cannot be overstated.

One easy-to-use accountability tool is the RACI model, or RACI matrix. (See Figure 4.2.) RACI stands for:

- **Responsible:** The *responsible* person is the person or team to whom the task was directly assigned. They work to complete the task or provide the actual deliverable. In a best-case scenario, every task should have at least one responsible person or team (Miranda & Watts, 2022).

- **Accountable:** The *accountable* person delegates and reviews the work involved in the project. Their job is to ensure that the responsible person or team is aware of the project expectations and completes the expected work in the agreed-upon timeframe. Each task should have only one accountable person. Having more than one accountable person creates confusion; people trip over each other with regard to who is *really* accountable (Miranda & Watts, 2022).

- **Consulted:** Individuals who are *consulted* provide input and feedback about the work being done for a project. They have a stake in the project's outcome because it could affect their own current or future work. It is ideal to consult these individuals before starting the work to ascertain their needs. It's also wise to check in periodically throughout the work to obtain their feedback on the status and outcome of the work. Not every task requires someone to be consulted. However, doing so provides an opportunity to solicit feedback from several possible stakeholders and allows for diversity of thought. The ideal balance is to solicit enough feedback to ensure the correct problem is solved, but not so much that it slows down the process. Seeking limitless feedback will stall any project or initiative (Miranda & Watts, 2022).

- **Informed:** These are individuals who should be *informed* about the progress of a project or initiative—whether things are going well or they're not going according to plan. However, they should not be consulted for feedback or input, and certainly not overwhelmed with the details of every task. They simply need to be kept abreast because the progress of the project might affect their own work at a broader level. Senior and executive leaders often fall into this category. These individuals should not be pulled into the weeds of a project—not only because they are high-level decision-makers but also because doing so means their feedback will overshadow that of consulted individuals (Miranda & Watts, 2022).

> Adopt an organizational accountability model and educate *all* leaders—not just nursing leaders—on how to successfully implement it. This will help to advance work that often stalls due to lack of accountability.

Responsibility Assignment Matrix – RACI

Role / Project Deliverable (or Activity)	Executive Sponsor	Project Sponsor	Steering Committee	Advisory Committee	Role # 5	Project Manager	Tech Lead	Functional Lead	SME	Project Team Member	Developer	Administrative Support	Business Analyst	Role # 4	Role # 5	Consultant	PMO	Role # 3	Role # 4
	Project Leadership					Project Team Member					Project Sub-Teams					External Resources			
Initiate Phase Activities																			
Request review by PMO	A/C	R/A				R/A	A/C		C										
Submit project request						R											A		
Research solution	I					R/A	A/C	A/C	C			C				C			
Develop business case	I	A/C	I	I		R/A	C	C	C			C				C	C		
Plan Phase Activities																			
Create project charter	C	C				R/A	C	C	C			C				C			

R- Responsible | A- Accountable | C- Consulted | I- Informed

FIGURE 4.2 RACI matrix (Smartsheet, 2023).

CONCLUSION

Healthcare is incredibly complex and is becoming more challenging every day. However, nursing doesn't have to remain stuck in this chaos. As nurses, we must break this cycle. It's up to us to find ways to create a future that allows nurses to get back to practicing nursing in a way that is safe, rewarding, and impactful. We must push back on the status quo and step up to drive not only new models of care but new models of nursing overall. It's imperative for all of us to push innovation along in our organizations to improve the chances it will stick. That's how we can facilitate the transformation that is needed.

REFERENCES

Advisory Board. (2021). *Hard truths for CNOs: The current and future state of the nursing workforce.* [PowerPoint Slides]. Advisory Board Nursing Executive Center National Meeting.

Hughes, R., Meadows, M. T., & Begley, R. (2022). AONL nurse leader competencies: Core competencies for nurse leadership. *Nurse Leader, 20*(5), 437–443.

Miranda, D., & Watts, R. (2022, March 25). *What is a RACI chart? How this project management tool can boost your productivity.* https://www.forbes.com/advisor/business/raci-chart/

The nine-box grid for talent management. (2017, September). In *R 2 wiki. Creative Commons.* https://r2.miraheze.org/wiki/File:9-Box_Talent_Management_Grid.jpg

Russell, R. G., Novak, L. L., Patel, M., Garvey, K. V., Craig, K. J. T., Jackson, G. P., Moore, D., & Miller, B. M. (2023, March). Competencies for the use of artificial intelligence-based tools by health care professionals. *Academic Medicine, 98*(3), 348–356. https://journals.lww.com/academicmedicine/Fulltext/2023/03000/Competencies_for_the_Use_of_Artificial.19.aspx

Smartsheet. (2023, January 17). RACI matrix. In *Wikipedia.* https://cio-wiki.org/wiki/RACI_Matrix

Weberg, D., & Davidson, S. (2021). *Leadership for evidence-based innovation in nursing and health professions* (2nd ed.). Jones & Bartlett Learning.

Weberg, D., & Mangold, K. (2023). *Leadership in nursing practice. The intersection of innovation and teamwork in healthcare systems* (4th ed.). Jones & Bartlett Learning.

> *"The day you are not solving problems or are not up to your butt in problems is probably a day you are no longer leading."*
>
> —Colin Powell

CHAPTER 5

Creating a Future-Facing Care Model

KEYWORDS

Care-delivery models, care team, staffing models, virtual nursing

This chapter attempts to provoke new ways of thinking and to encourage leaders to shift current care-delivery paradigms. It discusses topics including new care models, emerging roles, integrating technology into care delivery, and tech-enabled scheduling and staffing—and even touches on updating nursing education and training models.

OBJECTIVES

- Identify current nursing tasks that could be handed over to support team members or technologies and the plan to do so.

- Articulate the benefits and barriers of a virtual nursing model in your organization.

If you are not yet convinced that we need to transform nursing, I suggest you scan social media, healthcare journals, and news sites, or solicit the opinions of any nurse leaders you know. The results will rapidly become obvious: Nursing is in crisis.

Previous chapters discussed how we got here. Now, though, it's time to look forward. When you do, you will quickly conclude that we have no choice but to innovate our way out of this. There just simply are not enough human beings in the existing nursing supply pool, nor are there enough students in the pipeline to make up for ongoing and project-ed churn.

> The irony is, there are more nurses than ever. The problem is that they don't work in patient care. We must create practice roles to attract and retain nurses in patient care.

As discussed in Chapter 1, cur-rent data show we will be short 200,000 to 450,000 direct care nurses by 2025 (Berlin et al., 2022). The longer view is even more dire. According to the International Council of Nurses, by 2030, we will experience a deficit of 13 million nurses worldwide (International Council of Nurses, n.d.). This is a huge problem—especially if we continue to use nurses in the same manner and in the same roles as we do today.

> In 2021 the nursing pro-fession lost more than 100,000 people—"a far greater number than ever observed over the past four decades," say Auerbach et al. (2022).

Our challenge now is to future-proof nursing by attracting nurses back into patient-care roles. This means using nurses differently than in our current models. We must develop new roles, new care models, new training programs, and even new scopes and standards for our practice. To accomplish this Herculean task, all 4.3 million of us nurses must manage the transformation of nursing practice internally, while at the same time navigate the transformation externally among other disciplines and the general public. And we must do so as if we are on a burning platform: with a sense of urgency.

CHANGE STARTS WITH NURSES

Nurses are often not aligned in terms of what their issues are, how to prioritize them, and how to solve them. It is no secret that nursing has been a hotbed of incivility for many years. To move forward, we must be civil, collaborate, and get to work. Otherwise, we might not have a profession that we identify with in the future.

As nurses, we must define our problems, identify potential solutions, and implement them. We must continually iterate and use rapid-cycle change processes to problem-solve, to progress, and to end the chaos. This cycle will need to happen thousands—perhaps even tens of thousands—of times for us to come up with viable solutions for providing patient care and guiding our profession through this challenging time.

Chapter 1 discussed several unique and complex challenges facing nursing. These include problems with recruitment and retention, the workforce pipeline, faculty shortages, role creation, scope and standards, outdated licensure expectations, staffing, care-delivery models, nursing reimbursement, and nursing value and compensation models.

Our Image Problem

Ask any patient about their experience in a healthcare setting, and they undoubtedly share a story that involves a nurse. This helps explain why, as mentioned in Chapter 3, nursing has been voted "America's Most Trusted Profession" for 20 years in a row (Senior, 2022).

Unfortunately, however, we as nurses have not capitalized on the significance of this notable achievement. Indeed, we have squandered our opportunity to communicate why our role is important to health and wellness to the general public. Worse, many nurses have not aligned and mobilized around this message to solve our problems and dictate our future. The nursing profession has become fragmented and polarized.

In addition, even as nurses have been consistently voted "America's Most Trusted Profession," we have developed an image problem. This is because the public, other healthcare professionals, and—due to increasing specialization among nurses—even other nurses don't understand what we do. As a result, they don't recognize what we contribute to the healthcare ecosystem, let alone advance, amplify, and advocate for our work.

"You can't build an adaptable organization without adaptable people—and individuals change only when they have to, or when they want to."

–Gary Hamel

TODAY'S CARE TEAM

Before we can create a future-facing care model, we need some understanding of our current care teams. Staffing models are not one-size-fits-all affairs. They often include a mix of different types of nurses, such as registered nurses (RNs), advanced practice RNs (APRNs), licensed vocational nurses (LVNs), and licensed practical nurses (LPNs) for direct patient care. Staffing models also include various unlicensed personnel, such as nursing assistants (NAs), certified nursing assistants (CNAs), patient care technicians (PCTs), emergency medical technicians (EMTs), paramedics (EMT-Ps), medical assistants (MAs), and phlebotomists, as well as care coordinators and case managers. Finally, the care team might include respiratory therapists, physical therapists, occupational therapists, speech language pathologists, dietitians, and many other important members. (These are, of course, in addition to those people who provide leadership, management, and high-level oversight of planning, strategy, and finances, as well as those who supervise direct caregivers.)

Not long ago, in an attempt to increase the rate of nurses with a bachelor of science in nursing (BSN) degree, we encouraged the existing associate degree in nursing (ADN) workforce to go back to school to obtain a bachelor's degree. This decreased the number of nurses with only an ADN, and we even scaled back on LVNs/LPNs in hospitals. More recently, however, due to the extreme shortage of nurses, we have pulled many LVNs/LPNs back into inpatient roles and even called some out of retirement.

To prepare for the future, we must evaluate the composition of our care teams. This means assessing patient-care needs and identifying which roles are best-suited to provide the necessary care in any given department. Now more than ever, we need to clarify the benefit of each role, ensure that the right roles perform the right tasks, and at the same time, offload to technology tasks that humans no longer need to do.

Nurses today are routinely expected to perform tasks that do not require their level of skill or compensation. In fact, nurses spend 36% of their time on non-value-added work, amounting to $757,000 in nursing salaries on average per department per year (Storfjell et al., 2008). Moreover, they devote more time to support activities (56%) than to providing direct patient care (44%). Clearly, we are not working at the top of our licenses! This is obviously unsustainable—especially considering there aren't enough nurses to perform the tasks that only they can do. The obvious solution to this dilemma is not to reduce nursing headcount, but rather to delegate non-nursing tasks to unlicensed team members. However, these are in short supply too; between 2020 and 2021, the national average turnover rate rose from 27.5% to 35.5% for CNAs and from 28.6% to 38.1% for PCTs (NSI Nursing Solutions, 2022, p. 9).

Some organizations have resorted to hiring nursing students and even students in high school-level health science and STEM programs. This apprentice model has been a win-win, enabling these organizations to meet their staffing needs and providing students with useful clinical experience and confidence, as well as a modest income.

At the same time, we must consider how healthcare might evolve in the next five-, 10-, and 20-plus years, so the care team can evolve with it. This requires a deep strategic planning session with the nursing leadership team, physician leadership team, top-level executives, and local academic partners. This

session will involve using the
organizational strategic plan to
identify what service lines will
grow, what type of care will likely
be provided, the goal of that care,
where that care will occur, and
what roles will provide it. It also
involves developing a roadmap to
achieve the creation of new types
of care models and care teams, as
well as a pipeline to fill care roles.

> It's likely that the future
> will bring a shift from
> an inpatient-centric
> approach to healthcare
> to one that is virtual,
> outpatient, home-
> based, and preven-
> tion-focused. I talk
> more about this later in
> this chapter.

WORKLOAD-INTENSITY STAFFING MODEL

One important consideration is the "right" number or ratio of
nurses and non-licensed staff who render care to handle the
workload. Most healthcare organizations measure nurse productivity not in terms of care delivered, but by determining the
"right" number of nurses to perform care for a specific number
of patients—regardless of what type of care is needed. Unfortunately, this approach often devolves into a game of sorts, in
which organizations attempt to employ fewer nurses to deliver
care, but not *so* few that it isn't safe for the nurse or the patient.

Not surprisingly, from the point of view of the nurses who work
for these organizations, the resulting number is rarely enough.
In a 2022 survey by the American Nurses Foundation of 12,000
nurses, only 21% of respondents said that their unit had "the
necessary number of RN staff with the right knowledge of skills"
more than 75% of the time. (See Table 5.1 for additional survey
results.)

Table 5.1 Answer to the Question "How Often Does Your Unit Have the Necessary Number of RN Staff With the Right Knowledge and Skills?"

23% of respondents	< 25% of the time
27% of respondents	25–49% of the time
29% of respondents	50–75% of the time
21% of respondents	> than 75% of the time

(American Nurses Foundation, 2022)

This is a losing proposition for patients and nurses alike. Instead of taking this approach, it's far better to do the inverse: Consider how best to safely provide the necessary care in a particular unit, department, or population, and staff accordingly. This means shifting to a workload-intensity staffing model. In this model, the acuity and needs of each patient within a unit, department, and population, along with the total workload, drive the number of nurses who provide care.

> This is generally how physicians provide care, and for good reason. When physicians are pushed into using high-productivity models, evidence shows that patient care suffers.

In a workload-intensity staffing model, workload intensity— and by extension, a safer and more equal distribution of patient assignments and workload—is derived by evaluating patient acuity (Bacon et al., 2022). This involves the use of self-validating technology to harvest patient-related information from the electronic health record, including patient activity and the need to monitor tubes and drains, perform procedures such as dressing changes, and administer IV drips and medications. Sometimes the department may need more nurses than planned, while other times the acuity may indicate the need for fewer nurses.

In addition to allowing a more balanced approach to patient care, using electronic health records to assist with determining workload intensity allows for far more accuracy than paper-based, unreliable acuity systems of the past. It resolves age-old concerns around the inaccurate assignment of patient-care activities, often done in an attempt to reduce workload.

While this system is not perfect, and implementing it is easier said than done, it is far better than using an arbitrary number or ratio to determine how many patients each nurse should care for. It also addresses a top turnover trigger identified by nurses in survey after survey: workload and staffing issues.

Executives often oppose this approach, citing a significant increase in labor expenses as their reason why. But healthcare organizations currently spend outrageous sums on overtime, double-time, staffing bonuses, and traveling or agency nurses. Why not invest some of the money on loyal staff? It's possible to model the finances in such a way as to create cost savings for the organization *and* make the existing staff feel more valued. The message that all nurses must align behind is for organizations to "see nurses as an investment, not as an expense" (Kerfoot, 2022, p. 40).

AUTOMATING SCHEDULING AND STAFFING

Scheduling involves determining which staff will work on which dates and at what time. Generally speaking, automated scheduling tools, which simplify and streamline scheduling, have been around for more than 15 years. However, many healthcare organizations have not leveraged their potential. In fact, nurse executives frequently report that although their organizations have purchased a costly scheduling tool, not all nurses, or even nurse leaders, use it. Embracing these tools is critical, however, because they can manage scheduling much more effectively than their human counterparts. Ultimately, to maximize the benefits of these tools, organizations should require their use.

The most basic scheduling platforms enable staff to self-schedule by entering their availability using a computer or mobile device (keeping in mind, of course, that nearly all healthcare organizations are 24/7 operations that require nurses at night and on weekends). However, with appropriate rules, guardrails, and operating procedures in place, scheduling platforms can assist with the time-intensive job of staffing the organization with the appropriate number of clinical staff on any given day and shift.

More sophisticated (and costly) scheduling platforms also include tools like artificial intelligence (AI) and predictive analytics (PA). The best of these tools can also scan electronic health records (EHRs) in real time for keywords like *discharge, discharge planning,* or even *going home* to identify beds that will soon be freed up due to patients being discharged or transferred. They might even scan operating room (OR) data, data on scheduled procedural cases, and emergency department (ED) data to identify patients who will need a bed after their procedure is complete or after they've been admitted through the ED. Some of these platforms even integrate the scheduling function to predict how many nurses and non-licensed personnel are needed to staff a particular unit. This is where technology helps us and where the magic *really* happens!

These platforms can predict the census and throughput much more quickly and accurately than a human being can—assuming the data are up to date.

Different platforms perform differently and, by extension, provide varying degrees of confidence among staff. However, generally speaking, all of the staffing platforms that use artificial intelligence and/or predictive analytics currently attain 90-plus percent accuracy within an eight-hour window (approximately). Some platforms yield an even higher level of confidence on census predictions, however. In any case, as these platforms continue to "learn" the patterns within a given organization, their accuracy will improve, enabling healthcare organizations to become more efficient at patient placement, staffing, and throughput and to improve productivity by deploying employees to the units and departments that require them, even if only for a few hours. As organizations continue to adopt and optimize these platforms, they will begin to feel their true impact.

Often, these technologies are not more broadly used because they are costly. However, the cost benefits they deliver in terms of productivity and efficiency can vastly outweigh the financial investments associated with obtaining and operating these technologies when they are used as intended.

CREATING A POD-BASED MODEL

The goal is to leverage these technologies and the efficiency they bring to the point that they enable us to safely staff our units while we avoid stressing our staff in an attempt to meet budgetary goals. This can be tricky, however, because nurses are trained to meet the needs of specific patient populations.

One approach to overcome this limitation is to create *pods* (service line-based staffing) and assign a number of nurses and other caregivers with a given set of skills to each one. Each pod would then consist of a certain number of units and a larger pool of nurses, which could float to other units within the pod as needed. The unit-based managers work together to ensure adequate staffing across several units instead of just one or two. You can think of this as being like a mini specific float pool—for example, a medical/surgical pod might consist of three to six individual units, where each unit has a manager. Managers would be assigned to individual nurses as their point person to handle performance evaluations, assist with career planning, and address issues or concerns for the nurse. In turn the nurses work among any of the three to six units on any given shift. Since the pod is the larger work team, it reduces the anxiety associated with floating, promotes familiarity with a variety of care needs, and provides more flexibility for staff.

For example, suppose you have a medical/surgical unit with two, four, or even six pods. If the census on another unit rises, requiring additional staff, a medical/surgical pod with the necessary skill set could float to that unit instead of individual nurses. This helps improve the quality of care because each member of the pod is accustomed to working with the others. It also helps maintain a sense of community, strengthening the bonds within the pod while at the same time enabling members of that pod to connect with nurses in other units.

If your organization implements this model, you will want to adjust your hiring practices accordingly and communicate this in hiring interviews. The idea is to hire, orient, and train new nurses for a particular pod so the pod can float across multiple units. Be aware, however, that because pod nurses may be expected to have or acquire a more extensive skill set, they may require additional compensation.

> Flexibility in scheduling and staffing is a win-win.

HOSPITAL AT HOME

In recent years, due to rapid advancements in technology, we have learned that there is much we can do to treat patients outside the walls of hospitals. Although we were already exploring these possibilities before COVID-19, the pandemic was a key driver in their rapid adoption, as telemedicine consultations replaced many types of in-person visits during its first year.

Since then, a model called Hospital at Home (HaH) has gained momentum among organizations all over the country. With HaH, some types of inpatient acute care—generally of the medical/surgical variety—is provided to certain patients in their own home. While HaH was in use in small numbers and piloted in various facilities, the Centers for Medicare and Medicaid Services (CMS) waiver allows care for HaH patients in a narrowly defined category to be reimbursed at the same level as patients who receive care in a hospital. This was a catalyst for broad adoption of the HaH model. This waiver requires a physician, nurse practitioner (NP), or physician's assistant (PA) to conduct one telemedicine visit each day and a nurse to perform two in-person visits each day, with some minor differences in a few states. (A specially trained EMT-P may perform one of these visits instead of a nurse.) In addition, the patient is free to connect at any time to the HaH team using technology to express urgent needs or ask questions.

The HaH model can address capacity concerns for healthcare organizations. However, the model does still require organizations to employ nurses, which can pose a challenge for those with multiple vacancies or that have difficulties with recruitment and retention.

VIRTUAL NURSING

Virtual nursing care is a care-delivery model in which patients receive care from onsite direct care nurses supported by a virtual registered nurse (ViRN or VN) located outside the inpatient department, off-campus, or potentially even outside the state. VNs "support the team at the bedside to distribute the workload and provide greater satisfaction for both the patients and the nursing staff" (Ball, n.d.). Virtual nursing is not e-sitting, chronic care or mental health coaching, or observing e-ICU or physiologic monitors. It is nursing practiced in a different way. Areas of benefit for virtual nursing include 1) care team experience and outcomes; 2) patient experience, safety, and outcomes; and 3) cost and efficiency.

The onsite team typically consists of a charge nurse/supervisor and some combination of RNs, LVNs, LPNs, EMTs, MAs, CNAs, PCTs, and potentially others and may not be dissimilar from the current care teams. Virtual nurses do not replace onsite nurses, but rather supplement their work and streamline their workflows. Technologies to support remote patient monitoring—such as in-room sensors, cameras, speakers, and microphones, as well as clinical equipment—assist the VN and onsite team in caring for the patient.

> Virtual nursing offers nurses an opportunity to reimagine care models and the delivery of care—and to make nursing practice safer and more satisfying again. This exciting emerging role requires our urgent attention!

Ideally, VNs should have no less than three years of experience and must be competent in a multitude of skills, including team leadership, critical thinking, clinical knowledge, and interpersonal communication. They must also demonstrate proficiency in EHRs and master several different technology skills, all while working remotely (Cloyd & Thompson, 2020). The VN should preferably have a critical care or emergency department background. The VN often provides documentation assistance and can triage call lights and relay calls to the appropriate team member based on the level of prioritization to decrease call-light response time. In a clinical crisis or emergency, the VN can also provide rapid response support and use ACLS guidelines to guide the team through treatment protocols and administration of emergency care.

VN Responsibilities

VN responsibilities may include the following:

- Patient monitoring/safety
- Rapid response assistance/support
- New graduate nurse support through precepting on demand
- Orientation/onboarding assistance
- Real-time advisement
- Staff mentoring/education
- Patient education pre/post-procedure
- Medication teaching/reconciliation
- Provider rounding support
- Admission documentation (excluding assessment)
- Discharge documentation and teaching
- Triage and assignment of call lights
- Care coordination and communication with the care team (Schuelke et al., 2019, p. 323)

By taking on some or all of these (and other) time-consuming responsibilities, VNs significantly lighten the load of onsite nurses, freeing them up to spend more time with patients. This improves patients' perception of their care as well as patient outcomes.

If VNs are to be successful, they must be properly trained and prepared. This is not a role that all nurses should simply rotate through; it's a specialty that requires consistent practice and expertise. A successful virtual nursing program can be launched that has approximately 30–50% nurses who consistently work as virtual nurses and 50–70% who work both in the virtual nursing department and on an inpatient unit. The benefit of this type of staffing is that the nurses build collective trust and understanding. To this end, the American Association of Critical-Care Nurses has established practice standards for what they call the eICU. Similarly, the American Academy of Ambulatory Care Nursing has developed practice standards for telehealth nursing, which have resulted in the creation of a subspecialty of ambulatory care. The challenges of this role require strong nurses who develop expertise in this area; to that end, certification is likely forthcoming.

> Although the VN can coordinate patient care, due to proximity, the onsite nurse is typically the default nurse of record and primary decision-maker. If there are differing opinions, they are resolved through communication between the on-site nurse, the VN, and if necessary, the charge nurse/supervisor. (Clearly, in this model, communication is key!)

For more than a decade, Stanford has used a variety of virtual care models. In addition, Inova and Common Spirit have tested them for several years (Van Dyke, 2022, p. 13), and other systems are beginning to report positive outcomes as well. These models show promise in several metrics, including the following:

- Nurse satisfaction
- Physician satisfaction
- Patient experience (measured through HCAHPS)
- Hospital acquired conditions
- "Good catches"

- Improved mentoring/precepting experiences
- Shorter length of stay (LOS)
- Improved throughput and discharge times
- Increased retention
- Improved care efficiency (Schuelke et al., 2019).

It's not a question whether these models work; they do. In fact, organizations that have implemented virtual nursing have experienced a 20% reduction in their length of stay, a 35% reduction in nurse turnover, and a 24% reduction in contract labor (Advisory Board 2021, slide 28). However, we need much more data to demonstrate consistent outcomes and a strong return on investment.

> Discussions with organizations that are currently piloting or have implemented the VN role put the patient load for VNs between 12 and 20 patients per VN (depending on the tasks required). However, virtual care models are rapidly evolving, and there are no hard data to indicate how many patients a VN can safely oversee. This too requires study to determine the best virtual nursing model to deliver safe virtual nursing care.

In addition:

- Virtual care models can be scaled to additional inpatient units.
- These models are a great way to supplement the on-site care team. This can be particularly helpful in smaller or rural hospitals, which might not benefit from the same level of expertise as larger or urban hospitals.
- Constant observation and monitoring of patients by the VN (or the technology) lighten the load of onsite nurses, providing them with a sense of relief and enabling them to provide better, safer patient care (once they get past the sense of constantly being observed, that is).

- Virtual models represent a helpful recruitment and retention tool, particularly for drawing retired nurses back into the workforce and attracting nurses who have left the bedside due to the strenuous nature of direct patient care.

- Virtual care models are effective in post-acute care and long-term care settings—areas that are experiencing particularly severe nurse shortages.

- Virtual nursing delivered in home care scenarios is more closely aligned to monitoring and assisting with on-demand patient questions/care needs.

For more on implementing virtual nursing, see Chapter 8.

Virtual Sitters

A close sibling of the virtual nursing model is the *virtual sitter* model. Virtual sitters, also called *e-sitters*, have been around for more than a decade.

Some organizations have demonstrated cost savings of more than $1M by using virtual sitters. Moreover, organizations that regularly use virtual sitters generally do not report an increase in fall rates, and some even experience a reduction in falls. One organization experienced an overall 50% reduction in the patient fall rate after implementing virtual sitters (Advisory Board, 2021, slide 28).

These outcomes suggest that well-implemented and well-managed virtual nursing and virtual sitting models have strong potential to help mitigate the current workforce issues in healthcare. However, each organization should explore these new care models in a way that is safe and unique to their own risk profile.

For more on implementing virtual sitters, see Chapter 8.

CONCLUSION

The reality is that very soon, there will not be enough nurses to provide direct patient care. As nurses, it is important for us to lead the charge in developing novel care models, designing new roles, and providing leadership once deployed. We must give up non-value-added tasks and practice at the top of our licenses. And we need to focus on new opportunities to leverage our expertise as nurses. Directing new care-delivery models will require us to be nimble and push ourselves in ways that make us uncomfortable.

Evaluate your organization to build a business case for a virtual nursing model and redesign clinical workflows to promote role delineation through collaboration across the care team. Use this as a call to action, for if we cannot be courageous and bold by adopting new care models, our future as a profession may be in question. As nurses, this is our lane. This is our space. This is what we do best.

REFERENCES

Advisory Board. (2021). *Hard truths for CNOs: The current and future state of the nursing workforce.* [PowerPoint Slides]. Advisory Board Nursing Executive Center National Meeting.

American Nurses Foundation. (2022). *Pulse on the nation's nurses COVID-19 survey series: Workplace survey, June–July 2022.* https://www.nursingworld.org/practice-policy/work-environment/health-safety/disaster-preparedness/coronavirus/what-you-need-to-know/covid-19-survey-series-anf-2022-workplace-survey/

Auerbach, D. I., Buerhaus, P. I., Donelan, K., & Staiger, D. O. (2022, April 13). A worrisome drop in the number of young nurses. *Health Affairs.* https://www.healthaffairs.org/do/10.1377/forefront.20220412.311784

Bacon, C. T., Gontarz, J., & Jenkins, M. (2022). Transitioning from nurse-patient ratios to workload intensity staffing: What helps and hinders the change. *Journal of Nursing Administration, 52*(7–8), 413–418. https://DOI.org/10.1097/NNA.0000000000001174

Ball, J. (n.d.). *Virtual nursing: What is it?* American Nurses Association. https://www.nursingworld.org/practice-policy/innovation/blog/virtual-nursing-what-is-it/

Berlin, G., Lapointe, M., Murphy, M., & Wexler, J. (2022, May 11). *Assessing the lingering impact of COVID-19 on the nursing workforce.* McKinsey & Company. https://www.mckinsey.com/industries/healthcare/our-insights/assessing-the-lingering-impact-of-covid-19-on-the-nursing-workforce

Cloyd, B., & Thompson, J. (2020). Virtual care nursing: The wave of the future. *Nurse Leader, 18*(2), 147–150.

International Council of Nurses. (n.d.). *The global nursing shortage and nurse retention.* https://www.icn.ch/sites/default/files/inline-files/ICN%20Policy%20Brief_Nurse%20Shortage%20and%20Retention_0.pdf

Kerfoot, K. (2022, January/February). Leadership and the great rest: Rethinking possibilities for the future of nursing. *Nursing Economics, 40*(1), 38–41.

NSI Nursing Solutions. (2022). *2022 NSI national healthcare retention & RN staffing report.* https://www.nsinursingsolutions.com/Documents/Library/NSI_National_Health_Care_Retention_Report.pdf

Schuelke, S., Aurit, S., Connot, N., & Denney, S. (2019, October/December). Virtual nursing: The new reality in quality care. *Nursing Administration Quarterly, 43*(4), 322–328.

Senior, R. (2022, January 12). Numbers don't lie: Nursing most trusted profession again. *American Nurse Journal.* https://www.myamericannurse.com/numbers-dont-lie-nurses-most-trusted-again/

Storfjell, J. L., Omoike, O., & Ohlson, S. (2008, June). The balancing act: Patient care time versus cost. *The Journal of Nursing Administration, 38*(5), 244–249.

Van Dyke, M. (2022, May/June). The path of most resilience: Building a strong and fulfilled healthcare workforce. *Healthcare Executive.* https://healthcareexecutive.org/-/media/ache/healthcare-executives/mj22/he_mj22_downloadedition.pdf

"Insanity is doing the same thing over and over and expecting different results."

–Albert Einstein

CHAPTER 6

Leadership Tools for Transformation

KEYWORDS

Crowdsourcing ideas, design thinking, hackathon, innovation, nurse informaticist, work environment, workforce, workflows

This chapter covers tools and frameworks for leaders to assist in developing new approaches to care delivery and novel roles for nursing to thrive in a VUCA world. It discusses the importance of human-centered design; using the workforce, work environment, and workflow to frame ideation; and ways to harvest ideas such as the 25/10 crowdsourcing approach.

OBJECTIVES

- Explain how design thinking can identify solutions for challenges in nursing.

- Provide an example of an appropriate setting and topic to use the 25/10 crowdsourcing approach to solicit new ways to solve problems.

Transforming nursing will be difficult but not impossible. Fortunately, there are tools to help us challenge our own thinking and to explore new approaches to problem-solving.

As leaders, we are generally trained in conventional leadership thinking, and we develop traditional leadership, business, and management competencies. We rely heavily on evidence, as we should. But many innovative tools and frameworks lack the research to back them.

Despite our reliance on evidence, we must explore new collaborative approaches to problem-solving—collecting data or measuring impact as we do. The exploration of new intellectual frameworks is important to the success of our profession. It is at least in part because of our insistence on outdated models that we have found ourselves in our current dilemma.

Nursing 2.0

The result of a transformation in nursing is sometimes called *nursing 2.0*. Nursing 2.0 will be defined by a technological focus, new scope, new roles, and new standards of practice, as well as the continued digitization of healthcare. The transformation to nursing 2.0 represents an urgent opportunity for introspection into our profession. The future ahead is vast and unknown. There is no longer a status quo. We cannot go back to the way nursing was pre-pandemic. That time has passed.

A FRAMEWORK FOR TRANS-FORMATION

Nursing is a complex profession, and so are our problems. While some suggest that our current nursing shortage is *the* issue, it isn't. It's a symptom of deeper problems. Identifying these underlying problems is like peeling an onion. There are many layers. Often, solving one problem simply reveals another.

As we consider how to transform nursing and build a culture of innovation, it's important to keep the multi-layered nature of our challenges in mind. Using a framework to give shape to the various variables can help.

One such framework is the 3W Culture Framework. It identifies three general categories to clarify the thought process: workforce, work environment, and workflows. Using the 3W Culture Framework is a great way to organize discussions around problem-solving, planning, and executing a more innovative approach.

WORKFORCE

In the context of nursing, *workforce* is a broad term that refers to the nurses who provide direct care, act as leaders, and fill other nursing roles. The nursing workforce in the United States consists of more than 4.3 million registered nurses (RNs) and 670,000 licensed vocational nurses (LVNs; US Bureau of Labor Statistics, 2021).

The term *nursing workforce* is often used in a very broad, generalized way, as though it is one homogenous group. In reality, the nursing workforce is extremely diverse. There are many different roles and specialties within the nursing workforce, not to mention people of different ages and generations, genders, regions, certifications, educational backgrounds, tenures, and so on. It can be very daunting to account for them all when making changes.

WORK ENVIRONMENT

People often use the phrase *work environment* to refer to the physical place where people perform work. In the cases of nurses, the work environment is often thought of in terms of a unit, department, clinic, university, and so on. But a nurse's work environment is not just the place where they work. Like the word *environment* used by itself—which describes an ecosystem that includes both the physical environment and the people it contains—the work environment also encompasses the human beings within the place, including other nursing team members and leaders, other medical staff, ancillary staff, and even patients. Moreover, the precise meaning of the phrase work environment might differ depending on where a nurse's practice occurs and what type of work they do.

> The word *practice* can be confusing. To many it means to regularly perform an activity to improve one's proficiency. But in this context, the word's meaning is broader, referring to the work nurses perform, including patient care, leadership, research, academia, and so on. For example, my own areas of nursing practice are leadership and innovation.

WORKFLOWS

The term *workflows* describes the sequence of processes involved in the completion of a task or activity. This term has become popular in nursing over the last several years and is of particular importance in identifying ways to improve the delivery and outcomes of patient care.

Workflows are a very important part of any care-delivery model and have an enormous effect on how nurses deliver care. For this reason, nurses *must* be involved when an organization decides to change the care-delivery model or incorporate new technology that affects care delivery. No other discipline understands nursing workflows better than nurses do, just as no other discipline understands surgery processes like a surgeon does.

Framing Transformation

The following shows an example of using the 3W Culture Framework to organize thoughts around building a strong team.

Workforce

Build a competent and engaged team.

Focus on "hiring for fit."

Curate a diverse team of open-minded thinkers to collaborate around solutions.

Remove toxic people early to prevent them from negatively affecting the team.

Demonstrate the financial benefit (ROI) of an adequate team to safely handle the workload.

Work environment

Create a positive culture that people want to be a part of.

Frequently recognize your team and show that you value them.

Be flexible with scheduling.

Develop new roles and competencies.

Workflows

Leverage technology to improve safety, outcomes, and experience.

Remove man-made barriers.

Put "sacred cows" out to pasture (in other words, make the changes that are hard to make).

Use human-centered design to involve the direct-care team in defining and solving challenges.

USING DESIGN THINKING

Design thinking is a collaborative approach to innovating and problem-solving that focuses specifically on people. That is, it's a more human-centered approach. In healthcare, the goal of design thinking is to innovate and problem-solve while keeping in mind safety, outcomes, efficiency, and sustainability. Although many industries have embraced design thinking, healthcare has been slow to adopt it.

Design thinking involves five main steps:

1. **Empathize:** Think about the people who are experiencing the problem you are trying to solve or innovate around. Learn about the affected population, whether it's a specific patient population or a group of nurses. Explore the problem from their perspective. What is the issue through their lens? It might not be what you think. The best way to obtain their perspective is to include them in the conversation about the problem. Ask "why" five times to keep digging at the real problem, so you identify the *true* problem and not just a symptom (Penn Nursing, 2021).

2. **Define:** Using the information you gleaned in the previous step, define the problem, so you can ensure you're solving or innovating around the right one. What is the problem, exactly? How significant is it? How many people does it affect, and how often? What caused it? What do you expect to happen when the problem is solved? What are the predicted outcomes? What happens if the problem *isn't* solved? As you define the problem, compose a problem statement. This will assist you in the ideation phase (Penn Nursing, 2021).

3. **Ideate:** In this phase, you ideate possible innovations or solutions. *Ideation* is simply a type of brainstorming. It's all about blue-sky or bold thinking. Nothing is off the table. The objective is quantity, not quality. You want lots of ideas, not just the best ones; you can always filter them later. This phase calls for divergent thinking and diversity of thought. You need to cast a broad net instead of focusing on preconceived ideas or solutions. This is *not* the time to say any of the following: "That isn't how we do things here," "We can't afford to do that," or "We tried that a few years ago and it didn't work" (Penn Nursing, 2021).

4. **Prototype:** Build, assemble, or model a solution to the defined problem for testing. Note that the term *prototype* often refers to hardware or devices, but it can also refer to processes and systems (Penn Nursing, 2021).

5. **Test:** Test the prototype solution in the real world to see if it works. If not, try to ascertain what went wrong, what could have been done differently, and how the prototype might be improved (Penn Nursing, 2021).

The last three steps in design thinking—ideate, prototype, and test—are *iterative*. That is, you might perform them over and over, learning lessons and observing trends. Gathering information at each iteration is *vital*. In addition to serving as evidence (which is critical in healthcare), this can also prevent you from wasting time and resources exploring solutions that are unlikely to work.

> In healthcare, we often use the term *pilot* to describe the test phase. This is often stated as a small test of change.

A key principle of ideation is, "Fail fast and fail often." In other words, fail *before* you've invested fully in a solution. Then quickly learn from the failure, adjust your solution, and try again. It might be difficult for healthcare professionals to adopt this attitude. Our industry does not take any form of failure well. When we fail, we have a tendency to stay away from what failed instead of re-evaluating and trying again. This must change!

Penn Nursing offers an amazing open-source course called Design Thinking for Health, funded in partnership with the Rita and Alex Hillman Foundation, to guide you through the process of design thinking. You can find out more about the course here: https://designthinkingforhealth.org/the-course/.

> "The problem is often more important than the solution. It takes courage to pause and ask, 'Is this the problem we should be solving for?' Design thinking isn't always having an idea or an answer for everything. Tools grant us the ability to identify the right problem, explore the complexities of that problem, and co-create solutions with the greatest impact."
>
> —Brittany Merkle

Five Rights of Healthcare Innovation

As a nurse, you're no doubt aware of the five rights of medication administration: right patient, right drug, right route, right time, and right dose. A similar framework, the five rights of healthcare innovation, applies to innovating and problem-solving in healthcare, and it can be helpful during the design-thinking process.

The five rights of healthcare innovation are:

- Right problem

- Right solution

- Right time

- Right price (for scale and sustainability)

- Right education (to ensure safe and effective rollout; Clipper et al., 2019, p. 85)

While the term *right* may imply exact precision, the meaning in this case is closer to *best*, as in best solution and best timing.

The goal of this structured approach is to ensure that the team works to solve a specific problem affecting the unit, department, or organization, rather than developing "a solution looking for a problem."

HARNESSING THE HACKATHON

A hackathon (or similar event) can motivate and energize teams to create and innovate. Simply put, a *hackathon* "is an event that brings together experts and creates a collaborative environment for solving a certain problem" (Hackathon.com, 2021). You can think of a hackathon as any planned, collaborative, problem-solving event.

Hackathons began as a way to generate code, solutions, and ideas among computer programmers and IT professionals, but now they're done by people in all kinds of industries, including healthcare. Hackathons can range from large-scale, multi-day events with hundreds of people to more modest sessions of four to eight hours with 20 or so attendees. A hackathon, combined with design thinking, is a great way to kick-start the innovation process, solve problems, and foster a spirit of teamwork.

Hackathons take time to plan and execute. First, though, the problem should be clearly defined. This requires the assembly of a few people who are close enough to the problem to fully understand it to take a human-centered approach to pinning it down. Such an approach helps to establish the strategic direction of the hackathon and to ensure that it has guardrails and is not overly broad.

In addition, any relevant data and evidence should be gathered and shared in advance. This will fuel the ideation phase of the hackathon, steering you toward solutions based on the organization's data and current outcomes. The event won't be productive if everyone walks into it cold. It is not uncommon to plan sequential hackathons that build off each other to innovate different solutions that are like puzzle pieces.

Hackathons are most effective for smaller problems. However, they often fall short with problems whose solutions require sweeping change or transformation. Still, they can serve as a catalyst for a larger goal.

Organizations that can do some benchmarking and use evidence to guide the process have a better chance of identifying effective solutions.

With that in hand, you're ready to plan. As you do, keep these points in mind:

- **Time and date:** Select a time and date that allow for a high participation rate. For example, starting an event at 2 p.m. might not work due to the "hard stop" that many have, and starting at 7 a.m. might be similarly unfavorable to high attendance. Instead, consider starting an event at 10 a.m. to allow people to check emails before attending; that way, they'll be ready to pay attention and to focus on problem-solving.

- **Event site and space:** Choose an event space where participants can sit at tables facing each other, where there are walls for sticking notes and documenting processes, and where there's enough room to move about. This will promote high energy, which is conducive to thinking and sharing ideas. Also, snacks and beverages are always helpful to keep the energy levels high.

- **Supplies:** Bring a computer/laptop, screen, and projector; a whiteboard or easel; letter-sized paper or even butcher paper (for notes and diagrams); sticky notes (to document processes and map journeys); and markers and pens. Using a digital whiteboard can also be helpful.

  > Encourage participants to bring their own laptops to access data and literature and search for best practices.

- **Participant list:** Whom you invite depends on how many people are affected by the problem you're solving. For example, if you're trying to improve hospital throughput, you'll need to invite several participants from a variety of disciplines, departments, and shifts, such as house supervisors, emergency department representatives, charge nurses, case managers, a few physicians, a finance person, an informaticist, and so on. In contrast, if you're trying to overhaul pain scale documentation, you may want to invite a smaller, more targeted group. Be sure to include stakeholders like customers (internal or external, including patients if necessary) and staff with knowledge and expertise on data sources and reporting requirements to track outcomes. One more thing: Don't invite people who all agree. This leads to groupthink, *not* innovation!

> You need to strike a balance between having a large and unwieldy group and just enough people for the diversity of thought needed to generate creative solutions.

- **Pre-event materials:** Compile a packet of materials that clearly states the problem you seek to solve and contains any relevant data and evidence you have gathered in advance. Distribute this packet to all attendees well in advance so they can review it and be familiar with it before the hackathon.

> The more work you do in advance, the more likely it is you'll create an atmosphere for successful ideation during the hackathon event.

During the hackathon, the assembled participants should use a design-thinking framework to generate possible solutions to pilot (this discussion should reflect available resources and priorities) and define "successful" outcomes.

The *real* success of a hackathon becomes evident after the event. This is when evidence and data can be more rigorously reviewed, and the tough discussions take hold. As ideas take shape and pilots prove successful, you can scale the solution at an appropriate cadence. As you do, be sure to keep the group informed of both failures and successes to keep their interest. If anything, you want to over-communicate! This helps ensure accountability, which is extremely important if you want to prevent this from becoming just one more initiative in the initiative grave-yard!

> Hackathons are a great way to start the innovative thinking. But the work cannot stop here! This is simply where it begins.

CROWDSOURCING IDEAS

Too often, organizations look solely to leaders for innovations and solutions. This is almost always a mistake. As we work to transform nursing, asking for feedback is essential, and listening to all voices is crucial. Nurses are the foundation of patient-care delivery and the ones closest to the patient; as such, nurses must have input into solutions developed to streamline nursing practice and improve patient outcomes. Leaders cannot solve the problems of frontline nurses without their input.

Of course, there are the traditional methods to garner input, such as staff meetings, shared gover-nance councils, patient and family advisory groups, and workgroups, but more novel processes can also be employed. One such process is

> Bringing diverse groups together to solve problems is a great way to share different lived experiences and opinions, and it can help solutions be effective when properly planned and resourced.

25/10 crowdsourcing, developed using the open source Liberating Structures framework. This process enables "a large crowd [to] generate and sort their bold ideas for action in 30 minutes or less" (Liberating Structures, n.d., para. 1).

> The ideal space for 25/10 crowdsourcing is generous and allows for standing and moving about.

The 25/10 crowdsourcing process works like this:

1. Have everyone in your group write down their idea and one action step for an innovation or solution on an index card. (If you wish, you can pose a specific problem you want them to solve or allow each person to share their own problem.) (five minutes)

2. Let the group mill around, passing the index cards face down from person to person. No peeking (at least for a few minutes)! (three minutes)

3. Alert the group when time is up. (Music is a fun way to do this.) Then have them flip over whichever card is in their hand, read the idea on the card, quickly assign it a score from 1 (low) to 5 (high), and write that score on the card. (one minute)

4. Repeat steps 2 and 3 four more times.

5. After the last "milling and passing" session, have each person total up the score for whichever card they are holding. (Each card should have five scores.)

> The Liberating Structures website (https://www.liberatingstructures.com/) features many excellent open source tools, which are free to use.

6. Ask the group if anyone is holding a card with a score of
   25. If so, ask them to read the idea and the action step.
   Repeat this step for cards with a score of 24, 23, 22, and
   so on, until you have collected the 10 best ideas (five
   minutes). The top scores are the problems (and ideas) that
   deserve consideration for implementation.

LEVERAGING NURSE INFORMATICISTS

One resource that we should tap into more often is nurse informaticists. These talented individuals are often able to offer
unique solutions and best practices because they have access to
data that many of us lack. You should absolutely include nurse
informaticists in organizational discussions to tap into their
direct expertise!

The American Nurses Association Scope and Standards for
nurse informaticists empower them to "lead in the design and
promotion of useful, innovative information technologies that
advance practice and achieve desired outcomes" (American
Nurses Association, 2015, p. 9). We look to nurse informaticists to simplify keystrokes, modify fields in electronic health
records (EHRs), and build reports, but we often overlook their
real expertise: leading clinical design sessions and workgroups
to identify problems and work toward enhanced workflows that
include maximizing data needs to improve care outcomes and
nursing practice.

As we work to transform nursing practice and patient care,
we must foster new partnerships among direct care nurses,
nurse executives, other nurse leaders, and nurse informaticists.
Indeed, the American Organization for Nursing Leadership
(AONL) has created a guiding principle to establish a culture of

collaboration between the chief nursing executive (CNE), chief informatics officer (CIO), and industry partners (American Organization for Nursing Leadership, 2019).

Collaboration with nurse informaticists is particularly important with regard to EHRs and their outputs. Too often we load our dashboards and reports with information that we think is important, without questioning whether it actually drives better outcomes. The dashboards and reports that we use in our transformation efforts must harvest the input of the nurses who provide care. After all, they are the ones who know our workflows best.

On a related note, nurse informaticists can help us ensure that our EHRs collect the necessary information in the most efficient way. Many healthcare organizations add new fields to the EHR without eliminating redundant required fields. This further burdens nurses and other clinicians without improving the quality of the data we receive—meaning it does nothing to help us reach our real goal, which is improved patient outcomes. The bottom line is, collaborating with nurse informaticists helps ensure direct care nurses gain an understanding of and competency in informatics, which in turn helps all of us capture valuable data to solve problems and improve outcomes.

> Documentation should follow care practices, not the other way around!

"If you don't like something, change it. If you can't change it, change your attitude."

—Maya Angelou

CONCLUSION

This chapter presented frameworks, tools, and suggestions that may be new to you to help you innovate and problem-solve to improve nursing practice and patient outcomes. Chief among these was design thinking. Several industries have used design thinking for many years, and healthcare is now catching up. Solving our current challenges will require all of us to collaborate and share ideas. The most important thing is, don't be afraid to try. Even if things don't go as planned, you probably won't make anything worse! There is far more to be gained by us collaborating and innovating together than wishing for the "old ways" because we are uncomfortable doing things differently. Remember, hope is not a strategy! We are all in this together and are counting on each other.

REFERENCES

American Nurses Association. (2015). *Nursing informatics: Scope and standards of practice* (2nd ed.).

American Organization for Nursing Leadership. (2019, April 23). *Position paper: Nursing informatics executive leader.* https://www.aonl.org/sites/default/files/aone/informatics-executive-leader.pdf

Clipper, B., Wang, M., Coyne, P., Baiera, V., Love, R., Nix, D., Nix, W., & Weirich, B. (2019). *The nurse's guide to innovation.* Superstar Press.

Hackathon.com. (2021, December 22). *What is a hackathon?* https://tips.hackathon.com/article/what-is-a-hackathon

Liberating Structures. (n.d.). *25/10 crowd sourcing.* https://www.liberatingstructures.com/12-2510-crowd-sourcing/

Penn Nursing. (2021). *Design thinking for health.* https://designthinkingforhealth.org/the-course/

US Bureau of Labor Statistics (2021). *Licensed practical and licensed vocational nurses.* Occupational Outlook Handbook. https://www.bls.gov/ooh/healthcare/licensed-practical-and-licensed-vocational-nurses.htm

> *"The first rule of any technology used in a business is that automation applied to an efficient operation will magnify the efficiency. The second is that automation applied to an inefficient operation will magnify the inefficiency."*
>
> —Bill Gates

CHAPTER 7

Leveraging Technology on Our Terms

KEYWORDS

Ambient computer vision, care transformation, decisions support, digital transformation, documentation, emerging technology, metaverse, remote patient monitoring, robots, smart rooms, technology, virtual reality

This chapter identifies emerging technology to meet the needs of a healthcare organization and discusses the integration of technology into workflows to enhance outcomes, increase efficiencies, lower costs, and improve the safety of nursing practice. Its purpose is to encourage leaders to develop a working knowledge of emerging technologies and novel care-delivery approaches. Armed with this knowledge and new ways of thinking, nurse leaders can chart a new direction for nursing to thrive in a dynamic and chaotic environment.

OBJECTIVES

- Describe how technology can help us improve health equity.
- Explain how smart hospital rooms will improve patient care and nursing workflows.

A major theme of this book has been the impact of our current nursing shortage. There just aren't enough nurses to provide care—particularly if the role of nurses remains as it has been in the past. This fact offers a compelling reason to consider the use of technology in nursing and in healthcare as a whole.

Recent years have seen an increasing number of new technologies. These include artificial intelligence (AI), predictive analytics, robotics, natural language processing, ambient computer vision, and remote patient-monitoring systems. These technological tools have the potential to enhance safety for healthcare providers (including nurses) and patients. They can also act as a force multiplier, enabling healthcare organizations to deliver excellent care by supporting nurses (and other providers) who are stretched thin. Nurse leaders must be aware of these technologies and how they can help transform nursing.

Younger nurses are particularly open to and adept at using technology. A 2018 survey revealed that 74% of millennials reported that technology "makes their lives easier," and 53% indicated that they would give up their sense of smell over their use of technology (Rogers, 2018, para. 3).

DIGITAL TRANSFORMATION

The phrase *digital transformation* describes the adoption of new technologies to transform an organization or industry. For a variety of reasons, healthcare has been slow to adopt new technologies; the digital transformation of the healthcare industry is in its early stages. As a result, there are many aspects of healthcare that are ripe for digital transformation, such as:

- **Healthcare economics:** This includes metrics for cost and outcomes, reimbursement trends, and payer concerns.

- **Data streams:** These include EHR data, clinical trial data, imaging, biometrics, and even data from devices worn by patients and consumers.

- **Population-specific data:** These include census data, geographic data, demographic data, and public health records.

- **Informatics:** This includes data-driven algorithms, artificial intelligence and machine learning, data transmission systems, data security, cloud computing, and data storage.

- **Social, political, and governmental forces:** These include peer/social networks, information privacy rules, ethical standards, healthcare disparities, socioeconomics, disinformation/ misinformation, and regulatory requirements/changes.

- **Globalization:** This includes world health, disease prevention, economics, and the supply chain (Gannotta, 2022, p. 28).

The digital transformation of nursing practice and care delivery will be slow, intentional, and expensive. It will also require constant direction and monitoring. This is to ensure that:

- Technology functions as predicted.

- Information flows across systems as intended.

- Privacy and security remain top priorities.

- End users receive alerts and notifications as anticipated.

- Algorithms are routinely evaluated for safety, bias, and accuracy.

- The benefits are as expected.

To leverage emerging technologies safely and effectively, we as nurses must appropriately assess the capabilities and risks of each technology before implementing them in patient-care models. This requires design thinking—empathizing with the population experiencing the problem a technology is meant to solve, accurately defining the problem, ideating on the appropriate technological solution, developing a prototype, and testing the prototype, as discussed in Chapter 6.

Chief technology officers (CTOs), chief digital officers (CDOs), chief nursing informatics officers (CNIOs), and chief medical informatics officers (CMIOs) tend to play a leading role in much of this work. However, nurses and nurse leaders must be equal partners and also have a seat at the table, every step of the way. Otherwise, adopting new technologies will be neither effective nor sustainable. How can technology effectively solve a problem that pertains to the delivery of patient care if the nurses who provide that care are not consulted about that technology?

"Nursing needs to be at the table to inform design on innovations with digital health and technologies, including artificial intelligence, machine learning, robotics, and data science. Nurses are the data stewards and understand the context of care and clinical workflow better than any other clinician in terms of a comprehensive picture to inform technology development. Without understanding of context and content no amount of technology or data will help this industry—nurses as subject matter experts are critical to successful development."

–Dr. Susan McBride

Improving Health Equity With Technology

In addition to positively influencing nursing practice and improving safe care delivery, digital transformation could alleviate or even eliminate variables that contribute to systematized inequities in healthcare.

Consider the role that transportation plays in healthcare, specifically in prevention and treatment. Many of us take our ability to visit our provider for granted, but millions of people are unable to do this, simply because they lack access to transportation. For patients without reliable access to transportation, these visits simply don't occur.

Thanks to technology, we can facilitate provider visits and many other health services in different ways, such as via telemedicine. This mitigates the transportation issue, allowing equal access to preventive measures and treatment.

Of course, this assumes people have access to broadband internet service, which is required for telemedicine. At present, almost 19 million Americans lack access to reliable broadband internet service, making broadband internet access now a social determinant of health (Federal Communications Commission, n.d.). While technology like telemedicine is closing the health equity gap, the work is far from over.

EMERGING TECHNOLOGIES

Technology is rapidly improving and now supports many healthcare capabilities and enhancements. It can function as a force multiplier to supplement the current complement of nurses in any given department, improve patient safety, maximize patient care outcomes, increase cost-effectiveness, expand access to care, and streamline data collection (Clipper, 2022).

For the last several years, the integration of technology into patient care has occurred at a moderate but steady pace. However, it is likely to speed up out of necessity. This will enable us to deliver care more safely and accurately, monitor patients, provide and collect data for evaluation purposes, make better decisions, and sometimes even obtain an extra set of hands to assist. This section discusses some of the emerging technologies that can and will play a part in transforming nursing.

Everyone hates to hear it, but we don't have a choice. Here in the US, we must integrate technology into patient care to maintain current standards of wellness and to safely provide care to a country of more than 330 million people (a large percentage of whom are or will soon be members of an older demographic).

Remote Patient Monitoring

Remote patient monitoring (RPM) involves using technology to observe, interact with, and track a patient's vital signs and to transmit that data elsewhere for monitoring and analysis.

Historically, this occurred within a healthcare facility. That is, the patient was in a room within the facility, hooked up to machines that collected data on their vital signs, such as blood-pressure machines, temperature probes, EKG monitors, and oxygen saturation monitors. These data were transmitted somewhere in the same facility—for example, down the hall to a nurse's station or to an office building in the same city.

Now, however, the patient can be anywhere—in a different facility or even at home. Their data can be sent anywhere too—on the other side of town or even across the globe, in real time. And the data can include more than just vital signs. Cameras and microphones can be installed, or tablets can be deployed, to enable care providers to monitor patients through video and audio feeds and even communicate with them using a monitor.

As an offsite mechanism for observing a patient and their data in real time while the patient is in an entirely different location, RPM has nearly limitless applications for patient care. Indeed, it's the foundation on which most virtual care models are built. (We talked about these in Chapter 5 in our discussion of virtual nurses.) Since its inception, RPM has evolved at a fairly rapid pace and will likely become standard equipment in patient rooms across the continuum of care—including acute care, skilled care, assisted living, long-term care, home care, and more.

> RPM is one advancement in technology that has allowed us to so rapidly grow hospital care in the home setting.

The most common use for RPM is for e-ICU, virtual sitters, or e-sitters. E-sitters have been around for more than a decade. As this technology has improved, and as e-sitters have become more affordable, many healthcare organizations have begun using e-sitters in one way or another. A peripheral benefit of using e-sitters is that the remote monitoring equipment generates considerable data. Another is the ability of the monitoring staff member to intervene via direct voice interaction to prevent the patient from falling or wandering.

If your organization has not evaluated RPM technology in the past 12 months, it is worth evaluating again to ascertain whether advancements in this technology have made it a suitable supplement for the existing care-delivery model or whether it should be adopted for a virtual nursing model. As with all decisions around patient-care technology, nurses should be involved in the process of selecting RPM tools.

One way to implement RPM technology for e-sitting is to hard-wire specific patient rooms with a network-enabled camera and speaker to which an e-sitter can connect as needed and to move a patient you want to observe into one of those rooms. Moving patients in this way can be a hassle, however. Another option is to deploy a mobile device with a camera and microphone to the patient's room. The ideal (though most costly) option is to equip all rooms with this technology.

E-sitters are not 100% failproof. However, many organizations use them with high levels of success to reduce the use of sitters and to reduce fall rates. This is particularly true for organizations where there are not currently enough staff to provide essential direct patient care, let alone sitter services. An e-sitter is a great compromise.

Monitoring With Computer Vision

Humans aren't the only ones who can monitor patients and their clinical data in real time. Machines can, too, using monitoring equipment similar to that used with RPM, but with ambient computer vision. Ambient computer vision is "a field of artificial intelligence (AI) that enables computers and systems to derive meaningful information from digital images, videos and other visual inputs—and take actions or make recommendations based on that information," says IBM (n.d., para. 1). Critically, one action these systems can take is to send notifications to the appropriate person if they detect a predefined condition or some type of anomaly. "If AI enables computers to think, computer vision enables them to see, observe and understand" (IBM, n.d., para. 1).

In a healthcare setting, you can use mounted sensors to observe/monitor patients. Visual data captured by the camera are sent to computers on the cloud by way of a consistent internet connection; AI algorithms on those computers then analyze the data.

These algorithms "learn" acceptable limits for specific patient data points; the system then notifies the care team if these limits are exceeded. Such systems can also detect and are beginning to document when visitors and caregivers enter and leave, when the patient receives and eats their meals, the patient's position, and more.

> Ambient computer vision is a good example of a technology that acts as a force multiplier, performing an important task-based function that makes people more efficient to tend to other matters, while also improving patient safety and outcomes.

Building the AI algorithms needed for this process requires a tremendous amount of time and testing. Because patient safety cannot be compromised, it will likely take a while for these systems to be broadly accepted in the healthcare industry. Trust in these technologies can only be earned through the consistent demonstration of safe patient outcomes. Having said that, this technology is successfully being used by hundreds of organizations around the country and continues to get smarter and less costly.

Smart Hospital Rooms

Smart hospital rooms take the model described in the previous section even further. In addition to cameras, these rooms also include microphones and sensors on the walls and embedded in other equipment. For example, a monitoring device embedded in the patient's bed could detect the patient's position and movement. Similarly, a device in the patient's toilet could detect when the patient uses the bathroom and measure the volume of urine evacuated. And a device on the soap dispenser could record when hand hygiene is performed. All this information is then streamed to computers on the cloud, where AI algorithms analyze it for anomalies. Smart systems like these have a high potential to improve patient safety and patient outcomes (Sun et al., 2021).

The benefits of the smart room can be amplified through the integration of a real-time location system (RTLS). With these systems, a radio frequency identification (RFID) chip is embedded in staff members' ID badges. In this way, their movements can be detected by equipment in smart rooms and throughout the facility. So, when a staff member enters a room to deliver care, to give the bedside report during rounding, or for some other reason, that information is documented in the system.

The ultimate goal of the smart room is to improve patient care. One way it achieves this is by relieving human caregivers of the burden of monitoring patients and of documenting certain care activities. As an added bonus, these systems provide rich data that yield valuable insights—data that currently require tedious manual collection. All this frees human caregivers to spend their time on tasks that *can't* be automated. Just think how this could change the workflow and workload of nurses, as well as the rest of the clinical team. The possibilities are endless!

Much of this technology is already being tested and will be used on a larger scale in the very near future. Indeed, I expect smart hospital rooms to become the standard of care within the next decade (or however long it takes to replace aging equipment with more modernized technology), in part because smart technology can offload non-value-added work, assist with the documentation burden, and help compensate for the shrinking supply of nurses and other care team members.

Just as our homes are becoming smarter, learning how we live and what our preferences are to improve our daily lives, hospitals will become smarter, too. Imagine an Alexa built into every patient room. Smart rooms could be used for nearly anything; we are limited only by our imagination and access to capital funds.

> The introduction of the smart room is a paradigm shift. For the adoption of this technology to be effective, it will require a strong change-management process.

Simplifying Documentation

Any nurse or other clinician will tell you that documentation requirements for patient-related activities are quite literally the bane of their existence. Most modules used by care providers for clinical documentation purposes were simply tacked onto baseline systems meant to capture registration, financial, admission, discharge, and transfer data, making them cumbersome, unintuitive, and time-consuming to use. Compounding matters, nurses are often required to enter data that aren't terribly relevant. This renders the entire system less useful because it cannot generate good insights on bad data. (This is called *garbage in, garbage out*, or *GIGO* for short.)

Fortunately, there are tools that make documentation easier. For example, as discussed, we are at the beginning of having data generated by RPM devices, computer vision, and smart hospital rooms being automatically added to a patient's EHR instead of documented manually.

> These days, almost nothing seems more important than helping nurses reduce the burden of documentation. Every minute spent on documentation is a minute *not* spent on direct patient care!

Another useful tool is the concept of speech recognition technology (SRT). With SRT, a care provider speaks into a Bluetooth-enabled microphone or headset to add data to the EHR or other type of data-collection system, instead of typing it in or selecting options in different fields, through the use of a platform that enables the conversion of voice narration to written information. SRT is similar to dictation, but it goes one step further, using natural language processing to convert the resulting audio file to text. A recent study on the use of SRT revealed a 10% reduction in time spent on documentation with nursing shift assessment flowsheets alone (Everett et al., 2022). There are even platforms with artificial intelligence that can assist in the crafting of the documented narrative.

Physicians have used SRT for some time in the form of dictation, but this technique has not generally been adopted by nurses. This is likely because SRT platform providers have historically operated on a per-user/per-month subscription model, which can be costly. However, in recent years, many of these providers have shifted to enterprise licenses. These provide economies of scale, enabling nurses and other caregivers to adopt these tools. In the past, these types of expenditures were deprioritized or left completely unfunded. Today, however, the use of SRT is gaining traction in hospitals because it has become a relatively low-cost way to reduce the nursing workload and the time spent on documentation.

All this being said, it's critical that we address what items we require for documentation. That is, these technologies won't be as effective if we don't fix the underlying problems of our data-collection systems and collect only the data we need. Work on this has already begun, thanks to the rise of the CNIO. CNIOs have done a great deal to improve screen, data entry, and documentation workflows. In today's environment, simplifying these workflows can be a winning strategy when it comes to retaining nurses.

Decision Support

Nurses are so busy moving from one task to the next that their ability to safely process inputs and think critically can be disrupted. Each of these disruptions presents an opportunity for an error to occur. An inability to correctly process data inputs can cause a nurse to make the wrong decision, which could negatively affect patient care.

Decision-support technology that uses AI to process data inputs is proving helpful in providing safer practice alternatives for nurses making clinical judgments and decisions. Many of these inputs—such as physiologic monitoring data, lab results, nursing/provider notes, and vital signs—can be continually evaluated by AI, which can identify trends and patterns that may warrant quick intervention more quickly and accurately than we humans can. Examples of this type of technology include AI-based applications that evaluate patterns and trends in a patient's electronic health record (EHR). Some of these applications can identify and even predict sepsis and lethal arrhythmias. This capability is in use today, is growing steadily, and will improve outcomes, save lives, reduce costs, and make the delivery of care safer.

Robots

Service robots are another emerging technology in healthcare. Service robots work in place of a human to perform low-value, redundant, repetitive tasks. For example, service robots have worked in pharmacies for years as medication technicians, locating and retrieving bar-coded unit-dose medications for specific patients. This practice has proved highly successful—indeed, it has become an industry standard.

Service robots have evolved to the point that they can now be used by care teams to deliver medications, meal trays, and supplies to patient units. These robots typically operate by using a laser imaging, detection, and ranging (LIDAR) system for navigation and by "learning" the layout of their environment—for example, where the elevators are, where their retrieval and delivery points are, and so on.

> I'm talking primarily about service robots here. Surgical robots have been used to safely and effectively assist surgeons in the operating room for many years, and they continue to evolve, improve, and provide better patient outcomes in a growing number of surgical cases.

Nurses are learning that having a service robot on the care team can be very helpful. Recall from Chapter 5 that nurses spend more than one-third of their time on non-value-added work. Robots represent yet one more way to free up nurses who spend an inordinate amount of time hunting, gathering, and fetching to perform more critical tasks. It is highly likely that we will see many more non-value-added tasks in patient care areas assigned to robots in the near future due to workforce challenges (Clipper et al., 2018).

> In addition to providing assistance and support to the healthcare team, service robots also act as goodwill ambassadors, bringing a smile to the faces of patients, their families, and visitors who encounter them.

Virtual Reality

In addition to transforming how patient care is provided, we must reimagine how nursing education is delivered. This includes all forms of education, including school training, orientation and onboarding programs, professional development, and even annual competency assessments at their places of employment, including hospitals, clinics, and anywhere else patient care is provided.

One technology to assist with this is virtual reality (VR). VR involves wearing a special head-mounted display (HMD) with earphones and haptic (vibrating) hand controls to experience an immersive and dynamic virtual (simulated) environment.

VR is often employed for gaming, but it is also an excellent learning tool. In healthcare, students and professionals of all types can use VR to participate in simulations of extremely lifelike patient scenarios that require critical thinking, decision-making, and action, eventually hard-wiring into them the skills and techniques they're meant to learn. As just one example, we can run Code Blue training over and over, and even if we fail every time, we never harm a real patient.

The study of outcomes associated with VR education in nursing is in its early stages. However, other industries provide strong evidence to validate the impact of the use of VR in education. For example, the aviation industry has experienced a 50% reduction in human-error related plane crashes since the 1970s, when the industry began training all pilots using VR simulators (Pottle, 2019). More broadly, the use of VR for educational purposes has shown increased improvements in staff knowledge compared to traditional education methods that offer a less immersive educational experience (Kyaw et al., 2019). In addition, research has shown that VR can achieve a "large improvement in post intervention cognitive skill scores" compared to traditional learning, such as learning through textbooks and didactic lecture-based education (Kyaw et al., 2019, p. 7).

Unfortunately, VR for use in the healthcare education space is still somewhat costly, not because of the equipment required—indeed, HMDs have dropped in price—but because of the expenses associated with developing VR assets like clinical scenarios. However, it is possible to develop VR assets that can be shared and reused across organizations so they don't need to be created from scratch every time. You can even create templates for general scenarios that can be customized for each facility—for example, with different layout for units and patient rooms, different colors for scrubs, and other design and aesthetic features. It's all just a matter of preference and funding.

The Metaverse

A newer technological development is called the *metaverse*. Merriam-Webster describes the metaverse as "a highly immersive virtual world where people gather to socialize, play, and work" (Merriam-Webster, 2021). Mark Zuckerberg of Facebook, which has invested heavily in developing the metaverse, explains, "The defining quality of the metaverse will be a feeling of presence—like you are right there with another person or in another place" (Zuckerberg, 2021). It's a lot like VR, but more interactive. Dan Patterson at CBS News describes it as "a 3D social network." But "Instead of a profile, you have an avatar, and so do your friends. Instead of a news feed, you have social hubs where people gather to share news, gossip and play games" (Patterson, 2022).

According to Accenture (2022), the emerging metaverse has two functions: creating the "Internet of Place" and the "Internet of Ownership." This essentially means we will move away from using the internet as a place to find and source information to using it as a place to interact, create experiences, and produce information.

This metaverse is primed to use virtual reality as well as augmented reality and mixed reality (which combine computer-generated content with the real-world environment), especially as they relate to learning and socializing. Imagine the impact this will have on nursing schools, universities, professional associations and organizations, hospital orientation, and clinical team training. In fact, several universities are already exploring the metaverse with an eye toward establishing a campus type presence there in the future. The metaverse could also be useful for "in-person" conferences.

> The metaverse won't be for everyone. For example, older nurses might not be comfortable operating in the metaverse. However, younger nurses—particularly millennials and Gen Zers, who are more comfortable with technology in general— likely won't hesitate to adopt it.

When it comes to using the metaverse in a healthcare context, walk, don't run. Put some thought into the potential impacts and benefits of the metaverse on your patient population. The American Hospital Association (2022) offers these guidelines to help organizations be strategic in their approach to the metaverse:

- Become familiar with the role that gaming will play, including offering rewards, incentives, and recognition for those who change behaviors and improve outcomes.

- Consider an approach to a more person-centric mental health/behavioral health delivery platform to improve compliance and outcomes.

- The metaverse could offer a convenient, cost-effective online approach to personalized physical therapy.

- Evaluate the potential use of the metaverse for lifestyle and behavioral wellness programs such as weight loss management (American Hospital Association, 2022).

The metaverse will likely rapidly evolve, affecting healthcare in ways we cannot yet imagine. However, we will have to grapple with significant privacy, security, and safety concerns before we invest heavily in its use.

TECHNOLOGY IN CARE TRANSFORMATION

While some of these emerging technologies are already in limited use and are becoming more common, the real concern is how to make them interoperable (sharing data across platforms) as well as how to integrate them with care-delivery models. This requires working with informaticists, nursing staff, physicians, other interdisciplinary team members, and even patients using a human-centered design framework.

Transforming care-delivery models and integrating technology will inevitably reveal gaps in evidence to support the desired outcome. Don't let this become a barrier. Innovation requires iteration—ideating, prototyping, and testing over and over again. This inevitably results in the creation of evidence along the way.

Like all innovation, building a tech-enabled care model requires a clearly defined problem, well-thought-out goals—whether they involve streamlining workflows, improving efficiencies, providing decision support, or increasing safety—and strategically planned solutions (Clipper, 2022). The possibilities are endless, limited only by your budget and the willingness of your organization to change.

"

"The technology you use impresses no one. The experience you create with it is everything."

–Sean Gerety

"

CONCLUSION

To emerge from our current chaotic state, nurses must become both high-touch and high-tech. Fortunately, there are many technologies to help nurses deliver care more safely, accurately, and efficiently. These include remote patient monitoring, artificial intelligence, ambient computer vision, natural language processing, robots, virtual reality, and many others, not to mention technologies that we have not yet invented. As we consider these technologies, we must shift our thinking from "We can't" to "How might we?"

It's imperative to educate nurse leaders and direct care nurses about current and emerging technologies, including their functionality, associated risks, benefits, value proposition, and costs versus benefits. This will prepare them to evaluate these solutions to identify the ones most likely to meet their needs. If nurses are to lead in the transformation of nursing, they must be equal partners with the typical players in the technology space, such as the CTO, CDO, and CIO.

That's not all. Nurses must also be involved in the design and development of new technologies that impact nursing workflows. Too often, nurses are absent during the creation phase. And yet, they're the only ones who understand the steps involved in care-delivery processes, the sequence of workflows, and the strengths and weaknesses of these workflows, including profound inefficiencies.

Perhaps most importantly, when evaluating technology, the starting point must be, "What problem are we trying to solve?" A solution in search of a problem is a recipe for wasted time and money. For nurse-led teams to make the best decisions on technology, they require a clear goal, such as improving patient safety and outcomes, revamping cumbersome nursing work-flows, increasing nurse satisfaction and retention, improving cost and efficiencies of care, or reducing health inequities.

REFERENCES

Accenture. (2022). Digital health technology vision 2022. https://www.accenture.com/_acnmedia/PDF-178/Accenture-Digital-Health-Technology-Vision-2022.pdf

American Hospital Association. (2022). *4 ways to frame your future in the metaverse.* https://www.aha.org/aha-center-health-innovation-market-scan/2022-07-19-4-ways-frame-your-future-metaverse

Clipper, B. (2022, April). Going boldly ... into digitally enabled care models. *Nurse Leader, 20*(2), 141–144.

Clipper, B., Batcheller, J., Thomazl, A. L., & Rozga, A. (2018, December). Artificial intelligence and robotics: A nurse leader's primer. *Nurse Leader, 16*(6), 379–384.

Everett, M., Redner, J., Kalenscher, A., Durso, D., & Nguyen, S. (2022, Fall). Speech recognition technology for increasing nursing documentation efficiency. *Online Journal of Nursing Informatics (OJNI), 26*(2). https://www.himss.org/resources/speech-recognition-technology-increasing-nursing-documentation-efficiency

Federal Communications Commission. (n.d.). *Eighth broadband progress report.* United States. https://www.fcc.gov/reports-research/reports/broadband-progress-reports/eighth-broadband-progress-report#:~:text=Notwithstanding%20this%20progress%2C%20the%20Report,lack%20access%20to%20this%20service

Gannotta, R. J. (2022, April 1). Changes in the healthcare environment prompt leaders to think digitally. *Frontiers of Health Service Management, 38*(3), 24–30.

IBM. (n.d.) *What is computer vision?* https://www.ibm.com/topics/computer-vision

Kyaw, B. M., Saxena, N., Posadzki, P., Vseteckova, J., Nikolaou, C. K., George, P. P., Divakar, U., Masiello, I., Kononowicz, A. A., Zary, N., & Car, L. T. (2019). Virtual reality for health professions education: Systematic review and meta-analysis by the digital health education collaboration. *Journal of Medical Internet Research, 21*(1), 1–13.

Merriam–Webster. (2021, October 30). *What is the metaverse?* https://www.merriam-webster.com/words-at-play/meaning-of-metaverse

Patterson, D. (2022, March 3). *You've heard of the metaverse. Here's what it looks like.* CBS News. https://www.cbsnews.com/news/what-the-metaverse-looks-like/

Pottle, J. (2019, October). Virtual reality and the transformation of medical education. *Future Healthcare Journal, 6*(3), 181–185.

Rogers, S. (2018, October 23). Why millennials need VR. *Forbes.* https://www.forbes.com/sites/solrogers/2018/10/23/why-millennials-need-vr/?sh=46dc87836260

Sun, C. J., Fu, C. J., Morelli, J. D., & Levin, A. (2021). Improving bedside shift report and hourly rounding using remote surveillance. *Journal of Informatics Nursing, 6*(2), 16–22.

Zuckerberg, M. (2021, October 28). *Founder's letter, 2021.* https://about.fb.com/news/2021/10/founders-letter/

"For the times they are a-changin'"

—Bob Dylan

CHAPTER 8

Conclusion

Nursing is in a state of chaos. There are many reasons for this. A major one is that there are more nurses leaving the profession than there are nurses entering it due to a variety of complicated factors. As a result, there aren't enough people to handle the workload—and it's only going to get worse. The impact of this on patient care and on our profession as a whole is and will continue to be profound. Another is the complexity of the healthcare environment. A third is the toxic and sometimes violent culture in many nursing environments. This has resulted in widespread dissatisfaction, lack of engagement, and even apathy among nurses. Finally, there is COVID-19. Although the COVID-19 pandemic did not cause our current crisis in nursing, it has most certainly amplified and accelerated it.

Nursing is at an inflection point. It is clear we must use our current state of disruption to transform nursing. This will require solutions that are creative, innovative, and nimble. We must explore new care-delivery models that are nurse-led and patient-focused. This will mean developing new roles, integrating emerging technologies, or both, and iterating new ideas quickly on demand. We must also evaluate new approaches to building the workforce pipeline and to identifying and developing new leaders. Finally, we must find ways to accelerate our efforts through lobbying and through collaboration with professional organizations.

Transforming nursing will require a change in workplace culture. At a bare minimum, this means ensuring the work environment is free of violence, abuse, and incivility. Beyond that, it means developing a culture of innovation—one in which all nurses feel free to develop and share ideas to improve the workplace environment and the safe delivery of care.

Changing the workplace culture is some of the most difficult work that leaders do. Sweeping changes like these require leadership buy-in and commitment. Too often, though, attempts to change become nothing more than initiatives of the month. This won't do if we are to transform nursing. Accountability is key. On a related note, if our leaders are to be effective, we must alter their role to make it both more effective and more doable. Making nurse leaders more effective will require us to redefine key competencies of nurse leaders to include change management, innovation, transformation, systems thinking, relationship management, and optimizing influence. As for making the role of nurse leader more doable, this may mean reducing the span of control or making this work more flexible—for example, by offering job-sharing or remote-work options. Otherwise, we run the risk of accelerating the revolving door of leaders entering and exiting organizations.

Still, this is an exciting time to be a nurse leader. And fortunately, there are many tools and frameworks that leaders can use to facilitate innovation and transformation. This book introduced several of these. One of these was the 3W Culture Framework, which identifies three areas to consider when evaluating any solution: workforce, work environment, and workflows. Another was design thinking, which involves five phases to identify problems and possible solutions: empathize, define, ideate, prototype, and test. The book also discussed the critical importance of clearly defining the problem you want to solve in any change effort.

The transformation of nursing will require a transformation of a different kind: digital transformation. Digital transformation describes the adoption of new technologies to transform an organization or industry. The digital transformation of the healthcare industry is in its early stages. However, there are numerous emerging technologies that could revolutionize nursing practice, workflows, and instruction, as well as improve health inequities. These include telemedicine, remote patient monitoring, artificial intelligence and predictive analytics, ambient computer vision, smart hospital rooms, service robots, virtual reality, and the metaverse, as well as technological tools to assist with documentation and decision-making. Nurse informaticists can greatly assist in leveraging technology to tackle the documentation and data challenges facing your organization. These often hidden gems can do wonders to reduce the documentation burden and speed up the solution cycle!

As important as nurse leaders and other executives will be to the transformation of nursing, it is nurses themselves who must lead this charge. If we as a profession are not involved in the design and development of system and technological solutions to transform nursing, then we run the risk of being sidelined completely. We must read the clues in our current environment and spearhead a revolution to save nursing. There will be no formal invitation to nurses to save the nursing profession from obsolescence and irrelevance. But the chaotic state of healthcare demands our involvement. We must raise our voices—all 4.3 million of us—if we are to remain the connective tissue in healthcare.

It won't be easy. We will no doubt be hampered by budget constraints. Making big changes costs money (although it's often the case that *not* making these changes costs even more). That aside, to be successful, we'll need to work together toward a common vision—something we're not always great at. We'll also have to work with others outside nursing to identify new and effective ways to care for patients in an ever-changing healthcare environment. And we'll likely need to accept changes we've historically resisted, such as measuring workloads, adapting reimbursement methodologies, and developing new roles and team models. Then there's the issue of technology. As our numbers decline, technology will act as a force multiplier and will improve the safety and satisfaction of nursing practice. Therefore, nurses must become more open-minded about the role technology can play and take an active part in identifying and implementing technological tools to improve nursing workflows and practices. We as nurses must be high-touch *and* high-tech to ensure our continued success in this century and beyond.

The good news is that nurses are uniquely qualified to lead this transformation effort. In addition to being incredibly empathetic and intelligent, as well as gifted problem-solvers, many nurses exhibit positive deviance. It's what enables nurses to think critically and develop useful workarounds to expedite work on the fly. Oddly, although few nurses think of themselves as innovators, I believe our positive deviance makes us the greatest innovators of all. Indeed, you might say positive deviance is our superpower! We must scale this superpower to solve even larger problems.

Young nurses could prove especially critical in this effort, as they tend to be the most adept at technology and willing to change. To capitalize on this resource, we must support them in their learning and career goals. Many young nurses seek to advance in their careers more quickly than those who came before them. Rather than discouraging this, we must develop career lattices to facilitate it, and seek out more experienced nurses and nurse leaders who are willing to mentor these ambitious young nurses.

I hope this book has inspired you to jump into action and contribute to the transformation of nursing. It's a big job, and we'll need everyone's help to get it right! But don't become overwhelmed. Start at the micro level by becoming a force for change in your own unit or department. That's a great first step.

Be bold, and have the courage to #transformnursing.

With gratitude,
Bonnie Clipper

"You're off to great places, today is your day, your mountain is waiting, so get on your way."

–Dr. Seuss

Index